Jürgen Graf | Uwe Stüben

Handbook of Aviation Medicine
and Inflight Medical Emergencies

2nd Edition

revised and edited by Jürgen Graf

Medizinisch Wissenschaftliche Verlagsgesellschaft

Instructions for using this book

| Important statements – i.e. sources of errors, dangers when evaluating a situation or practicing a scheme

Specific medicinal considerations to special features on board, especially medical reasons to continue the flight versus a nonscheduled landing

Background information worth knowing (i.e. scientific data) to different statements in the text

Jürgen Graf | Uwe Stüben

Handbook of Aviation Medicine and Inflight Medical Emergencies

2nd Edition

revised and edited
by Jürgen Graf

Medizinisch Wissenschaftliche Verlagsgesellschaft

Prof. Dr. med. Jürgen Graf
Medical Director and Board Chairmen
Klinikum der Johann Wolfgang Goethe-Universität
Frankfurt
Theodor-Stern-Kai 7
60596 Frankfurt am Main

Prof. Dr. med. Uwe Stüben
Geschäftsführer der Deutschen Akademie
für Flug- und Reisemedizin
Lufthansabasis
60546 Frankfurt am Main

MWV Medizinisch Wissenschaftliche Verlagsgesellschaft mbH & Co. KG
Zimmerstraße 11
D - 10969 Berlin
www.mwv-berlin.de

ISBN 978-3-95466-239-5

These publications are listed in: Deutsche Nationalbibliothek
Detailed bibliographical information is available via internet http://dnb.d-nb.de.

Project management: Anna-Lena Spies, Berlin
Editorial office: Monika Laut-Zimmermann, Berlin
Translation (1st Edition): Petra Illig, Anchorage, USA
Layout and typesetting: eScriptum GmbH & Co KG – Digital Solutions, Berlin
Printing: druckhaus köthen GmbH & Co. KG, Köthen

Reply and complaints to:
MWV Medizinisch Wissenschaftliche Verlagsgesellschaft mbH & Co. KG, Zimmerstr. 11, D - 10969 Berlin,
lektorat@mwv-berlin.de

Preface to the 2nd Edition

Commercial aviation transports about 3 billion people per year between countries and continents in ever larger jet aircrafts which theoretically can each accommodate up to 839 persons (e.g. in Airbus A 380–800 with maximum seating configuration, current cabin layouts can take on approximately 535 passengers). With modern long-haul and ultra-long-haul aircraft distances of up to 19,000 km are covered and thus non-stop flight times of more than 18 hours can be achieved. At the same time innovative technologies and design techniques have been introduced in commercial aviation; to save weight and thereby increase the performance and range while reducing fuel requirements, the Boeing 787 – the so-called 'Dreamliner' – is the first manufactured aircraft in the era of modern wide-body aircrafts where the fuselage consists largely of carbon-fiber reinforced plastics. Moreover, the pressurization of the cabin is significantly different from any other commercial aircraft currently in use: instead of applying 'bleed air' from the compressor stages of the jet engines this is produced by independent turbine engines, integrated into the hull of the fuselage underneath the wing roots, in order to generate the necessary atmospheric pressure in the aircraft cabin. Among other companies, Boeing advertises that the new aircraft design allows a lower cabin pressure altitude. For example, the atmospheric pressure within the aircraft cabin at cruising altitude which is usually around 2,400 m (approximately 8,000 ft) is reduced to 1,800 m (6,000 ft). This would – as explained in this book in detail – lead to a higher oxygen partial pressure during the flight and thereby promises to passengers and crew members more comfort at that time. For people with a hypoxia-sensitive disease, pulmonary limitations or difficulties with pulmonary gas exchange, this may lead to a reduction in risk for the occurrence of e.g. a stroke or heart attack during the flight. To what extent these developments can compensate for any present rise of medical incidents in commercial aviation, is yet unclear.

The proportion of acutely and chronically ill passengers, elderly and frail people as well as passengers with physical and mental limitations and the need of support services at the airport or on board has increased steadily in recent years. Due to anti-discrimination regulations in global aviation industries, all airlines and airports face significant challenges to accommodate all passengers with their personal needs due to physical or mental restrictions.

For dealing with medical incidents on board, both the new generation of aircraft as well as the demographic, health and legal changes and the resulting composition of the passengers' community all provide a further challenge: in larger aircrafts with more and presumably even sicker passengers and longer flight times, the probability that a medical incident may occur during the flight increases statistically. Simultaneously, the chance is greater for affected passengers and/or patients that doctors or other healthcare professionals who provide primary care should then be among them on such flights.

In order to furnish helping doctors on board with the necessary aeromedical, technical, and organizational background for the handling of medical emergencies on board, the first edition of the 'Handbook of Aviation Medicine' was published in 2011.

The rapid development in recent years, both in commercial aviation and related regulations, as well as in the field of emergency medicine made a thorough revision and new edition of the handbook necessary. Although much energy has been put into the correction of errors and the valid presentation of regulations here, one must not forget that the framework in air transport as well as in medicine is continuously changing and we therefore have to adapt our knowledge and derived actions constantly. Thus, although all information and recommendations within this handbook are reviewed to the best of our knowledge, they have to be applied with caution when it comes to individual patients and any specific emergency situations.

We hope that with this book we achieve support not only for crews and potentially ill passengers on board requiring medical aid, but also for physicians on board that have had a chance to review some of the specifics when it comes to commercial air transportation.

We wish us all an enjoyable, trouble-free flight and a safe return!

Prof. Dr. Uwe Stüben, Prof. Dr. Jürgen Graf
Frankfurt am Main, February 2016

Preface to the 1st Edition

Air transportation has developed at an extremely rapid pace for the past 50 years. While it was possible only for the wealthy to undertake a journey by air a few decades ago, today flight is affordable for nearly everyone.

Passenger air travel has consistently increased by 5% to 7% each year in the past decade; today approximately 2 billion people travel by air every year. With the development of the so-called "no frills" airlines in the last few years, flights of thousands of kilometers are possible at costs comparable to travel by road. For those who are flexible and are timely in their purchase of an airline ticket on the internet, today the world can be explored at relatively low cost. This is such a fascinating development for the individual traveller, that he often forgets that he can find himself in an entirely foreign culture and climate within a few hours, potentially leading to medical care and standards to which he is not accustomed in the event of illness. As a rule, this price-conscious tourist, who travels as cheaply as possible, and who, as a last-minute tourist does not even know where he may vacation tomorrow, usually does not engage in proper medical preparation for his trip. The expectation that medical standards found in one's home country are equivalent to those in developing countries brings thousands of tourists into financial difficulties every year when faced with the need to repatriate as quickly as possible to avoid the treatment typical of the developed country in which they find themselves. General practitioners as well as travellers are often unaware of the risks that may lurk regarding travelling long distances in the event that prior medical conditions worsen or injuries occur while on vacation, necessitating returning by air ambulance or commercial flight. If the traveller has not considered these risks prior to travel and did not procure travel insurance, then the shock and financial burden is quite great when faced with the refusal of the airline to transport the passenger, necessitating air ambulance or services from a repatriation organization.

This book is based on the authors' many years of experience as aeromedical practitioners at Deutsche Lufthansa, making medical clearance decisions regarding injured and ill passengers on a daily basis. It should help physicians and travellers understand the peculiarities and stresses of air travel in order to avoid the pitfalls and stumbling blocks when dealing with medical problems. If the provided recommendations and the regulations are followed, nothing should stand in the way of an uneventful trip.

In this light, I wish all readers wonderful flights and a healthy and happy trip home.

Prof. Dr. med. Uwe Stüben

Contents

Contents

Contents

Contributors

This Edition is based upon contributions from the original German edition „Taschenbuch Flugmedizin und ärztliche Hilfe an Bord" and "Handbook of Aviation Medicine and Inflight Medical Emergencies".

Dr. med. Andreas Gabel, Ettlingen
I.5 Patient transport by commercial aircraft
III.5 Cardiovascular emergencies on board
III.6 Pulmonary problems

Dr. med. Jan Gebhard, Leiter Lufthansa AeroMedical Center, Hamburg
III.3 Motion sickness
III.4 Fear of flying
III.10 Choking from foreign body aspiration on board (adults)
III.11 Colics
III.13 Problems and emergencies with children

Dr. med. Günther Kaul, Straubing
I.4.2 Semi-automated external defibrillator (AED)
I.4.3 Oxygen
I.4.4 Satellite telephone – Medical hotline
II.9 Disabled passengers
(co-author Uwe Stüben)
III.7 Unconsciousness/seizures on board
IV.1 Who may do what during CPR?
IV.2 Resuscitation – Adults
IV.3 Resuscitation on board – Infants and children
V.1 Documentation of medical emergencies on board

Dr. med. Matthias von Mülmann, Lensahn i.H.
I.1 The aircraft cabin
I.2 Turbulence and vibration
I.3 Risk of onboard injury

I.4 Onboard medical equipment
I.4.1 Emergency medical kits
II.1 Medications, checklists, travel medicine
II.2 Time zone changes
II.3 Problems of adjustment to pressure changes (barotrauma)
II.4 Traveller's thrombosis
II.5 Medical conditions and flight fitness
II.6 Pregnancy and flight fitness
II.7 Travelling with children (medical advice)
III.1 Medical diversions (co-author Günther Kaul)
III.2 General considerations regarding medical emergencies (co-author Günther Kaul)
III.8 Intoxication from alcohol, medications or drugs
III.9 Food poisoning
III.12 Injuries and burns
V.2 Doctor-On-Board programme

Prof. Dr. iur. Wolf Müller-Rostin, Bonn
I.7 Legal aspects of medical assistance on board commercial aircraft

Prof. Dr. med. Uwe Stüben, Geschäftsführer der Deutschen Akademie für Flug- und Reisemedizin, Lufthansabasis, Frankfurt a.M.
I.6 Regulations regarding the transportation of ill passengers
II.8 Travelling with toddlers (legal regulations)

Chapter IV has been fully revised by Dr. med. Christina Jaki (Stuttgart) and Prof. Dr. med. Jürgen Graf (Frankfurt am Main).

I

Basic principles

1 The aircraft cabin

1.1 Cabin pressurization

There are many fundamental differences between air travel and ground transportation. Today's modern jets fly at altitudes between 30,000 and 40,000 feet. The Concorde, which is no longer in service, attained an altitude of 48,000 feet. The jet engines currently in use function effectively in thin air, and therefore at higher altitudes. Future developments are expected to not only meet, but to exceed these altitudes. Suborbital flights will subject crew and passengers to entirely new demands.

The atmospheric conditions found at flight altitudes places humans into an environment that is not survivable without appropriate technological measures. The temperature is around –60° Celsius, and the atmosphere is extremely thin and therefore does not contain enough oxygen for respiration. The consequence would therefore be death by freezing and hypoxia. The remedy is provided by cabin pressurization, which began in commercial aviation in the 1950s with piston engine airplanes, and which subsequently became the technical standard in jet engine aircraft. Information regarding the function of the pressurization and air conditioning systems in modern commercial aircraft is therefore presented here. On the one hand, these physical and physiological conditions set the prerequisites for the determination of the aeromedical fitness of passengers, and on the other hand, they set the limitations for care and emergency treatment on board, as well as for the feasibility of transporting ill passengers in commercial aircraft.

Modern airliners are powered by jet engines, where 80% of the thrust comes from the so-called bypass system and 20% through the engine exhaust. This makes for more economic utilization of fuel and also is more efficient, quieter, and produces less pollution. In principle the air is drawn in and compressed, causing it to heat up. This occurs over several stages, and eventually kerosene is injected and ignited. The exhaust contributes only a small portion of the generated thrust. The majority is created by the fan and secondarily by the turbines, which generate and deliver the greater portion of the propulsion in the bypass system. No combustion occurs here, and the cold bypass stream that is generated helps dampen engine noise.

The second of three compression stage of the turbine, in other words, before fuel injection occurs, is where the so-called "bleed air" is tapped and fed to the cabin pressure/air conditioning system. Compression heats the air to about 220° C. This is where the first problem arises, which is the low relative *humidity* in the cabin. Air at flight altitude is quite dry – only about 3% relative humidity, and this is reduced even further by the effects of compression. After subsequent cooling, the cabin air becomes extremely dry. It is sent to the individual seat rows through a distribution system, and flows in a far-reaching laminar flow along the cabin walls. In wide-body jets with two aisles, it also flows down from the luggage compartment areas, is eventually collected at the floors and exhausted through a collection system. Depending on the number of passengers on board, a portion of this air is drained through an outflow valve at the rear, while another portion is cleaned through a highly effective filtration system and admixed with fresh air (bleed air). This so-called *recirculated air* brings cabin humidity up to 8–15%. As an example, a Boeing B747-400 with a cabin volume of 1,900 m³ provides an air exchange of 16 to 24 times per hour, depending on the numbers of passengers.

The effective cabin *air pressure* is not, as is often quietly assumed, the same as at sea level. Due to technical reasons, such as enhanced structural requirements and thus greater weight, the cabin altitude is kept between 1,800 m and 2,450 m. Therefore the cabin pressure is lower than at sea level. The International Civil Aeronautical Organization (ICAO) allows a maximum cabin altitude of 3,000 m – a level that is not normally achieved in today's modern aircraft. It is only approached when the destination airport is at a higher altitude, such as La Paz in the South American Andes Mountains.

This choice of cabin altitude was not reached arbitrarily, but rather guided by physiological principles. The healthy human organism tolerates an altitude of up to 3,000 m (about 10,000 feet) quite well by adaptation, and therefore problems are not expected.

A relevant point is that the cabin pressure naturally does not remain constant, but changes according to flight level. After takeoff, it declines incrementally to a minimum, only to rise again through descent to landing. Pressure changes can also occur at cruise altitudes (see Fig. 1).

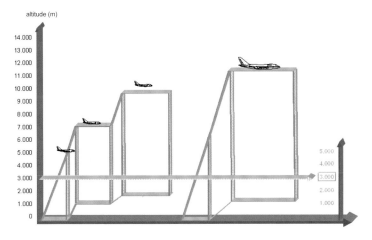

Fig. 1   Cabin pressure vs. outside pressure

In the past, cabin pressure was set manually by the flight engineer, while today it is automatically regulated in relation to the outside pressure. This technique is more comfortable for the passenger, as it allows for smoother transitions. Nonetheless, in certain situations dependent on air traffic control specifications and flight profile requirements, cabin pressure can be rapidly adjusted by hand. Theoretically it is possible to construct the cabin and air conditioning system in such a way as to maintain a pressure equal to that on the ground. However, this would lead to higher weights due to increased structural requirements, thereby reducing range and load capacities and resulting in higher ticket prices.

A brief mention regarding *temperature* should also be made. Cabin temperature is controlled independently for different sections of the aircraft. The Airbus A340, for example, has six zones in which individual temperatures can be set. Depending on passenger load, electromagnetically driven valves can mix compressed, re-cooled air from the so-called *pack* with diverted warm air. At this point it is worth mentioning a phenomenon that often causes concern and worry for laypeople thinking that there may be a fire on board. After landing in hot, tropical areas with high humidity, the cabin is cooled for comfort. By virtue of this cooling of moist outside air, which is brought in through the air conditioning system, thick plumes of vapour can be seen coming out of the overhead gaspers.

In keeping with the *"fail safe principle"*, which means that for each system in the airplane there is at least one (often two, three or more) redundant system in the event of malfunction, there are two, or even three, air conditioning systems. Therefore even in the event of a rapid decompression, a sudden loss of pressurization is safeguarded against while an appropriate lower flight level can be attained to minimize health hazards.

1.1.1 The gas laws

There are three main gas laws that are important to mention when discussing environmental conditions in an aircraft cabin. They are listed below in order of significance for aviation medicine:

1. Boyle-Mariotte law
2. Dalton's law
3. Henry's law

The Boyle-Mariotte gas law

This law states that the volume of a gas (or a mixture of gases) at a constant temperature and humidity is inversely proportional to the pressure to which it is subjected. Gas pockets in the human body are usually composed of air with a high moisture content, so that the vapor pressure of 47 mmHg must be subtracted, resulting in this equation:

$$\frac{V_2}{V_1} = \frac{pG_1 - pH_2o}{pG_2 - pH_2o}$$

Air is a mixture of gases in which the pressure declines logarithmically, and at an altitude of about 5,000 m is reduced to half. As a rule this pressure change is not dangerous, but neither is it irrelevant as it can cause significant discomfort as well as pain. All passengers are affected similarly. Particular predisposing factors that are not manifested at sea level can lead to painful symptoms through pressure differences, such as eardrum anomalies or problems in the nasal sinuses.

Dalton's gas law and oxygen delivery

Air is a mixture of nitrogen, oxygen and minute amounts of a variety of noble gases. According to its percentage of the total, each gas exerts its proportional share of the total pressure according to the following equation:

$$P_{ges} = P_1 + P_2 + P_3 + P_4 + P_5 + \ldots + P_n$$

Again, this assumes constant temperature and humidity. As before, normal travellers are subject to this effect, and it carries particular significance with regard to oxygenation. As the total pressure decreases, so does the partial pressure of oxygen with a corresponding reduction in *oxygen saturation of the blood*. This process, too, does not run linearly, but logarithmically. The human body has the ability to compensate to a certain degree (see Fig. 2), basically up to a pressure altitude of 3,000 m; above that, compensation is time-limited or not possible at all.

Furthermore, the laws of gas diffusion must be taken into consideration. This purely physical process is passive and always runs in the direction of falling pressure gradients until equilibrium in both compartments is reached. The medium in which this process takes place plays no role. Media can be gaseous, liquid or solid and do not necessarily have to be subdivided by membranes – although this is, of course, always the case in biology. The speed of diffusion depends not only on the concentration gradient, but also on the thickness and permeability of the membrane and the size of the molecules of the respective substance(s). Another factor is the diffusion surface area. Certain lung diseases create thickened alveolar membranes and reduced surface areas, resulting in a further reduction of arterial pO_2 and oxygen saturation (see Fig. 3).

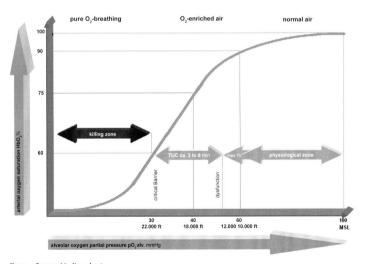

Fig. 2   Oxygen binding chart

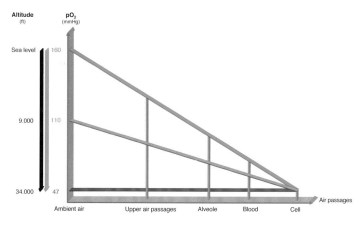

Fig. 3 Oxygen saturation chart: Oxygen pressure reductions in MSL (green) and at 2450 ft (orange); Ambient oxygen pressure in cruising altitude of 34.000 ft or above (red). MSL = Mean Sea Level

The effect of *Dalton's law* is very important with regard to aeromedical evaluation in that diseases of the cardiovascular system, the lungs, and the blood are significantly impacted. It describes the problems associated with hypoxia – of which there are four types. They all have the same outcomes, but arise from different causes.

Hypoxic hypoxia is caused by insufficient oxygenation in the inspired air, when the partial pressure is too low, as it occurs with increasing altitude. This does not normally happen in commercial aviation as the aircraft is always pressurized to a comfortable level. In the event of a decompression, oxygen masks drop from above the seats and the aircraft rapidly descends to a safe pressure altitude. Other complicating factors are diseases of the gas exchange system in the lungs, such as thickening of the alveolar membranes or a reduction in gas exchange surface areas often found in patients with emphysema.

Anaemic or *hypovolaemic hypoxia* is caused by an insufficient O_2 transport capacity of the blood. Primary anaemia or blood loss is first on the list. Toxic gases such as carbon monoxide or substances such as nitrates or sulphur compounds lead to similar effects due to their high affinity for haemoglobin.

Histotoxic hypoxia is the result of a disorder of oxygen utilization within the cell, such as cyanide poisoning. But also narcotics and alcohol significantly impair oxygen utilization.

Circulatory (stagnant) hypoxia is caused by a circulatory failure, which can arise from a variety of sources.

Henry's gas law

Gases dissolve in liquids and body tissues. The amount of gas dissolved in solution varies directly with the pressure of that gas over the solution or within the tissues. This gas law is described in the following equation:

$$\frac{P_1}{P_2} = \frac{Q_1}{Q_2}$$

The emphasis in this case is primarily on the tissues and only secondarily on fluids, therefore it should be pointed out that different tissue structures have different affinities to various gases – especially to nitrogen.

Henry's gas law plays a minor role in aviation medicine. It explains the mechanism of decompression illness of divers (Caisson's disease). Its effects are not seen often in daily practice.

1.2   Humidity

Due to the extremely low humidity of the air at flight levels processed by the pressurization system in commercial aircraft, cabin air is relatively dry. After an hour of flight, the humidity drops to a level between 8 and 15%. There is a linear relationship between the humidity and the number of passengers on board (see Fig. 4). In a fully occupied B747-400, a maximal humidity of 15% can be achieved. Even the proportion of recirculated air plays a significant role. The greater the amount of incoming fresh air, the lower the humidity. Humidity is generated exclusively from the recirculated air component, which is cleaned by HEPA filters and mixed into the air circulation. This has a direct influence on the level of comfort.

The mucous membranes of the mouth and nose dry out, generating a sensation of thirst which increases fluid intake. However, kidney function does not initiate a diuresis, but rather the fluids shift to the extravascular space of the lower extremities due to the relative immobility and mild hypoxia.

Simultaneously, the dry air affects the conjunctivae, resulting in nonspecific irritation and a foreign body sensation in the eyes. This is why it may be a good idea to instill artificial tears. Contact lens wearers should consider taking extra precautionary measures.

1.3   Temperature

In contrast to many air conditioning systems, the technical solution for temperature control is not a significant problem. Because the passenger compart-

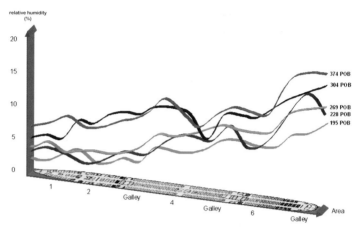

Fig. 4   Relative humidity, and distribution in the cabin (POB = Passengers On Board)

ment is divided into many (up to eight) zones, temperature regulation can usually meet the demand. Nonetheless, there are also some limitations. The sizes of the sections are dependent on construction requirements and cannot be altered. The class sections do not necessarily conform to these zones. It is therefore entirely possible that the temperature zone in the spacious business class may carry over to the more densely packed economy class. A dilemma may then arise: If the area that is less densely occupied is kept comfortable, it may become too warm for the other zones and vice versa.

With this in mind, it is recommended that one should wear warm clothes while flying – even when travelling to tropical countries. This is all the more important because many flights, especially to the Far East and Southern Africa, are night flights. Appropriate clothing promotes better quality of sleep when considering the lower body temperatures that are experienced during night and early morning hours.

Incidentally, the cargo hold is air conditioned as well.

1.4   Extraterrestrial radiation

In general, extraterrestrial radiation is not a problem for the normal passenger. A flight from Frankfurt to the west coast of the United States, such as to Los Angeles, results in an exposure of 30 µSv. A flight to Japan via a polar route results in 62 µSv and a flight to Rio de Janeiro in 18 µSv. The different doses are caused by the variability of the protective magnetosphere of the Earth. It is less in the polar regions than in the equatorial latitudes.

The European radiation regulatory agency UTA recommends a maximum of 20 mSv for travellers over a period of 5 years, and not more than 4 mSv annually.

Caution is recommended for first trimester pregnancies. There is no data regarding early fetal damage. In Germany, maternity protection law prohibits further flight duty for flight attendants and pilots during pregnancy.

1.5   Special exposures

A variety of other influences can negatively affect comfort during long flights, even though they may not be related to health issues. Some of these factors have been eliminated with technical solutions; others are prohibited by law.

First and foremost, *smoking on board* has been an issue in the past. Despite partitioning into the corresponding sections and elaborate air conditioning, the problem was never satisfactorily solved for the adjacent sections. Only since the regulatory agencies issued a general smoking ban for all flights the complaints have ceased.

A similar situation existed with regard to *ozone loads* until ozone catalytic converters were introduced. Particularly in the spring and on North Atlantic routes, ozone can project deeply into the atmosphere. By flying through these ozone layers, it can be brought into the cabin through the air conditioning system, which does not contain any measuring or warning devices. Typical complaints include: dry cough, retrosternal burning, pronounced irritation of the eyes, etc. The problem was solved in 1995 with the introduction of ozone catalytic converters which convert this gas into harmless O_2.

Periodically, the public is confronted with reports that the air conditioning system of airplanes *promotes the transmission of infectious diseases*, such as tuberculosis, to other passengers. For many reasons these reports are not accurate; in individual cases transmission does occur – but by other routes! By virtue of the technical construction of the air conditioning system, the air flow routing, the highly efficient filtration systems (HEPA) and the extremely dry air, transmission via this route is ruled out. However, it is quite possible that the previously ill person can disperse infection in his or her immediate vicinity by way of droplet contamination, or by moving through the aircraft such as to the lavatory or the galley. In reported cases, the recommendations of the World Health Organization (WHO) are followed and those passengers who were in the area where droplet spread could have occurred, namely two rows in front of, beside and behind the infected passenger, are notified. The HEPA filters are so effective that even particles the size of a virus are eliminated. A number of independent research institutes and organizations have repeatedly studied and verified this on several flights.

In new aircraft, as in newly constructed buildings, a variety of solvent residues may emanate from plastics, glues and carpets. These concentrations are well within the limits set by the regulations on *maximum allowable concentration (MAC)*, and generally only play a short-term role as they dissipate after a few flights due to the high air exchange rate, and only occasionally recur after repairs and maintenance.

Carbon dioxide accumulates in the area of the galley more than in other compartments of the cabin. The source is dry ice used for cooling the food and beverages. Here, the regulatory limits can definitely be reached, but are not exceeded. There is no concern regarding the passenger.

The aircraft is disinfected and disinsected by an exterminator at regular intervals during its lifetime in order to avoid a pest infestation.

1.6 Space and mobility

Flight times are getting longer, and some routine commercial flights are up to 18 hours in duration. With few exceptions, and according to seating class, the space limitations result in various types of discomfort – some of which could be considered as health issues. The relative immobility leads to tensions in the back muscles, and pain in the spinal column, pelvis and leg musculature. The large joints can become painful and stiff. This is due to *sitting in one position for a long time*. These complaints are transitory in nature. The lower legs can become swollen with secondary circulation disturbances. In persons who are particularly predisposed, *deep vein thrombosis* can develop, with the possibility of pulmonary embolism in individual cases.

> Particularly at risk are individuals with varices and/or other risk factors such as obesity, nicotine use, genetic disposition, or use of oral contraceptives.

At this point, a brief mention of a **legal perspective** should be made. Periodically passengers attempt to make the airline liable for health problems that develop during flight to obtain compensation for injury or pain. There are several unequivocal rulings in German case law which have determined that travelling inherently carries a risk. This means that many things in daily life have an associated risk and that the individual must take this into account.

2   Turbulence and vibration

Turbulence, vibration, and other unfamiliar factors can not only provoke motion sickness, but also fear of flying.

For those who are predisposed to motion sickness, it is best to reserve seats in the aircraft's middle section. The sensations are much less pronounced here than in the front or rear of the aircraft.

Additionally, long-range aircraft with long tail sections have a tendency to side motion. The recommendation by the flight attendants to always have the seatbelt securely fastened during flight should always be followed and is meanwhile mandatory! In rare cases at high altitudes, significant turbulence can be encountered which is not predictable, and can lead to very severe motions of the aircraft. Altitude changes of 1,000 m within a few seconds are entirely possible. Every year, such situations occur and often lead to serious injuries such as bone fractures among passengers and cabin personnel.

In serious cases of *motion sickness*, antiemetics in the form of medicinal chewing gum or transdermal patches are a remedy. The former has the advantage of rapid onset within a few minutes, while the latter must be applied prior to flight. Sedatives or alcohol are not suitable approaches to treatment.

3   Risk of onboard injury

Time and again, air travel gives rise to preventable injuries, often caused by disregarding onboard procedures. This particularly applies to *the placement of overly heavy hand luggage in the overhead bins*. The possibility of these bins opening during turbulence, and luggage falling down onto passengers, unfortunately always exists and is entirely unpredictable. Many injuries occur in this manner!

The recommendation by the flight attendants to always *have the seat belts securely fastened* and to remain seated is often not observed, especially by frequent fliers.

4   Onboard medical equipment

The contents of the medical kit on board a commercial aircraft are mandated by regulations; however, these serve only as minimum standards. In Europe, they are determined by EASA (*European Aviation Safety Agency*). Since these specifications represent European law, they must be implemented through national law in the individual countries. The airlines have the liberty to go beyond these requirements. The medical service of *Lufthansa German Airlines AG,* for example, has been procuring advice from leading emergency physicians and anesthesiologists on which medical equipment, instruments and medications to supply.

> **Important notice:** The following tables and figures only represent the current situation at the time of the writing of this handbook, and are subject to change.

The aircraft of *Lufthansa German Airlines AG* are equipped with the first aid materials described in the following, exceeding the legal requirements. All drugs include package inserts with instructions on use and information regarding indications and contraindications as well as effects and side effects. Additionally, the trade name and generic name are stated. Furnishing of the medical equipment can only be performed at the home bases, Frankfurt, Hamburg and Munich, and replacement of depleted medications and materials overseas or at other German airports is not possible. Therefore, in certain, rare circumstances the complete supply range may not be available.

There are three levels of medical emergency equipment:

1. *Cabin Attendant Medical Kit* for minor medical problems
2. *First Aid Kit* particularly for injuries
3. *Doctor's Kit for* severe medical situations

The contents are arranged in different *modules*. Depending on the illness, each module can be opened separately. This facilitates a general overview, and at the same time, the entire equipment needed for a specific situation is readily at hand.

For *cardiac* emergencies, a semi-automatic defibrillator is available on every flight.

4.1 Emergency medical kits

4.1.1 Cabin Attendant Medical Kit

The Cabin Attendant Medical Kit provides first aid medications for those small urgencies that occur on a daily basis (see Fig. 5). The flight attendant must be confident in its use and in a position to administer the contained medications responsibly without relying on additional guidance. The con-

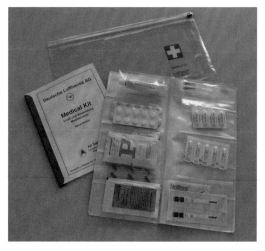

Fig. 5   Cabin Attendant Medical Kit

tents of the Cabin Attendant Medical Kit depend on the flight profile, i.e. continental vs. intercontinental routes (see Tab. 1 and 2), while the number of kits on board varies according to aircraft type.

Tab. 1 Cabin Attendant Medical Kit contents (Cont version)

Preparation	Substance	Unit
Steryl Kit (Plaster)		Pieces
ASS Hexal (500 mg)	Acetylsalycylacid	Tabs
Nasal drops Otriven (0.05%)	Oxymetazoline	Phiole

Tab. 2 Cabin Attendant Medical Kit. Contents of the additional intercontinental version

Medical Supplies/Product name	Substance	Unit
Burns- and wound gel 20 g	Lidocaine	Tube
Buscopan dragee	Hyoscine Butylbromide	Dragee
Buscopan supp.	Hyoscine Butylbromide	Supp
Imodium Akut dragee	Loperamide	Dragee
Paracetamol 250 mg supp.	Paracetamol	Supp
Magaldrat	Aluminium Phosphate	Sachet
Protagent eyedrops	Povidone	Phiole
Reusable Thermometer		
Vomacur dragee	Dimenhydrinate	Dragee

List of contents Medical Kit

4.1.2 First Aid Kit

The First Aid Kits are bandage kits (see Fig. 6 and 7). Its contents are designed to take care of minor and medium injuries which can occur on board a commercial aircraft (see Tab. 3). The injuries range from harmless sprains and bruises to lacerations and fractures.

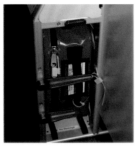 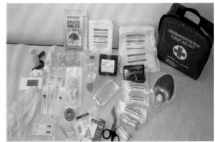

Fig. 6   First Aid Kit (storage space)   Fig. 7   First Aid Kit (content)

The First Aid Kit also contains a portion of the *intravenous fluids*, which cannot be accommodated entirely in the Doctor's Kit. First Aid Kits are identically packed on board of all aircrafts. Number and storage depend on the type of the aircraft.

Tab. 3   First Aid Kit contents

Medical Supplies/Product name
Gauze swab (Aluderm) 7.5 cm x 7.5 cm
Bandaging pack (Aluderm), medium
Bandaging cloth (Aluderm), 60 cm x 80 cm
Bandaging cloth (Aluderm), 80 cm x 120 cm
Clauden Gaze 2 cm x 5 m
Bandage triangular
Disposable gloves, unsterile, size 8 1/2
Thermometer, disposable
Fixation tape for permanent venous catheter
"Hansaplast Elastic", 1 m x 6 cm
Infusion instrument
Eye rinsing liquid, Tima-oculav, 250 ml
Jonosteril, 500 ml electrolyte solution for infusion (pouch)
Contaminated sharps container
Clip plaster
Dress shears

Medical Supplies/Product name
"Leukofix" adhesiv tape, 5 m x 1.25 cm
Garbage bags (set)
"Octenisept" desinfectant for wounds (Phenoxy ethanol)
Pincette
Respirator with O_2 connector
Splint
Plug for permanent venous catheter
Permanent venous catheter 18G, 20G and 22G
Tourniquet
Clamps for bandaging
Bandaging elastic 4 cm x 6 cm
Bandaging elastic 4 cm x 8 cm
Alcoholic swabs
List of contents First Aid Kit
First Aid book
Liability waiver
Datalink

4.1.3 Doctor's Kit

The Doctor's Kit (see Fig. 8 and 9) is an *emergency medical kit* which is provided to voluntary physicians in order to treat *life-threatening conditions*. It is to be used *exclusively by physicians* and is not intended for use by laypeople. The in-

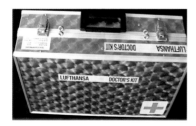

Fig. 8 Doctor's Kit (outside)

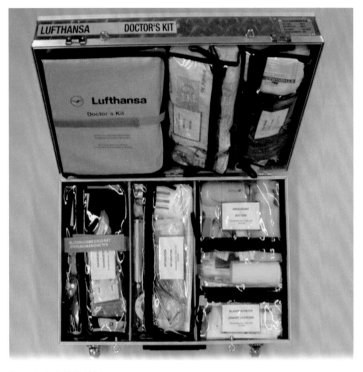

Fig. 9   Doctor's Kit (inside)

struments and assortment of medications are chosen so that the kit can be used by any doctor in accordance with his or her skills and knowledge. Specialty items were consciously avoided in order to reduce intimidation.
The Doctor's Kit contains materials according to the type of emergency:

- Six different modules (see Tab. 4 and Fig. 10–15)
- A set of ampoules (see Tab. 5)
- A plastic pouch with additional prescription drugs (see Tab. 6)

Tab. 4   Contents of the Doctor's Kit

Medical Supplies/Product name	Generic name
Modul: Intubation	
Syringe 10 ml, disposable	
Tracheal tubes CH 3; 4; 5; 6; 7.5	

Medical Supplies/Product name	Generic name
Disposable gloves size 8 1/2 (non sterile)	
Tracheal adaptor size 3	
Lube (Instillagel 6 ml)	
Laryngoscope	
Laryngoscope blade size 2.3	
Adhesive tape 5 m x 1.25 cm	
Magill forceps	
Cotton gauze bandage 6 cm	
Modul: I.V. Fluids	
Antiseptic alcohol swabs	
Disposable gloves size 8 1/2 (non sterile)	
Fixation patch for venous cannula	
I.V administration set for grafity infusion	
Jonosteril Freeflex solution 500 ml	Electrolyte solution
Gauze swab 7.5 cm x 7.5 cm	
Adhesive tape 5 m x 1.25 cm	
Closing – Stopper	
Cannula with injection port 18G, 20G, 22G	
Modul: Urinary catheder	
Aqua dest. Ampoule/10 ml	
Catheter, urine, disposable CH 12 + 14	
Syringe 10 ml, disposable	
Antiseptic liquid (Braunol 2000 30 ml)	Povidon Jod
Disposable gloves size 8 1/2 (sterile)	
Lube (Instillagel 6 ml)	
Drape sheet 45 x 75 cm	
Aperture drape sheet 45 x 75 cm	

Medical Supplies/Product name	Generic name
Gauze swab 7.5 cm x 7.5 cm	
Disposable Forceps	
Urine pouch 1000 ml	
Modul: Suction	
Suction catheter CH 14, CH 18, CH 22	
Disposable gloves size 8 1/2 (non sterile)	
Hand Held Portable Suction Unit	
Modul: Ventilation	
Resuscitator with Reservoir	
Transparent mask for babies size 0	
Transparent mask for children size 1	
Resuscitation mask for children Gr. 2	
Resuscitation mask for adults Gr. 5	
Disposable gloves size 8 1/2 (non sterile)	
Oropharyngeal airways size 0, 2, 3, 4	
Disposable oxygencatheter, Nose	
Disposable catheters + Tubes with connector	
Modul: Diagnostics	
Sphygmomanometer – manual	
Disposable gloves size 8 1/2 (non sterile)	
Finger pulse oximeter	
Single-use clinical thermometer	
Blood sugar test set	
Scissors	
Tourniquet	

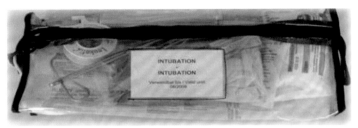

Fig. 10   Module intubation

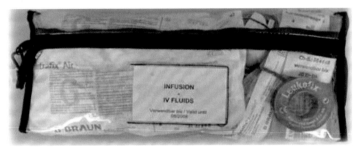

Fig. 11   Module infusion

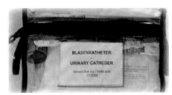

Fig. 12   Module urinary tract catheter

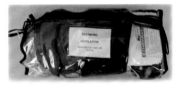

Fig. 14   Module airway

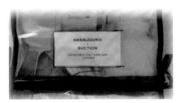

Fig. 13   Module suction

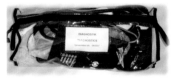

Fig. 15   Module diagnostic

Tab. 5   Medications in Doctor's Kit – ampoules set

Medical Supplies/Product name	Generic name	Unit
Adrenalin 1:1000 Jenapharm ampoule/1 ml	Epinephrinhydogentartrat	Ampoule
Akineton ampoule 5 mg/1 ml	Biperidenlactat	Ampoule
Amiodaron-ratiopharm ampoule 150 mg/3 ml	Amiodaron-HCl	Ampoule
Aqua pro injectione ampoule 5 ml	Aqua destillata	Ampoule
Aspirin i.v. ampoule 500 mg	Acetylic salicylic acid	Ampoule
Atropin ampoule 1 mg/ml	Atropinsulfat	Ampoule
Beloc i.v. ampoule 5 mg/5 ml	Metoprololtartrat	Ampoule
Berotec N 100 dosing aerosol	Fenoterolhydrobromid	Spray
Bronchoparat ampoule 10 ml	Theophyllin-Natriumglycinat	Ampoule
Bronchospasmin ampoule 0,09 mg/1 ml	Reproterol	Ampoule
Buscopan ampoule 20 mg/1 ml	Butylsopolaminiumbromid	Ampoule
Cetidem	Cetirizin	Tabs
Diazepam Ratio 10 mg/2 ml	Diazepam	Ampoule
Dormicum ampoule 15 mg/3 ml	Midazolam	Ampoule
Glucose 40% ampoule 10 ml	Glucose	Ampoule
Ebrantil 50 mg ampoule/10 ml	Urapidil	Ampoule
Haldol-Janssen ampoule 5 mg/1 ml	Haloperidol	Ampoule
Heparin-Natrium-5000-ratiopharm	Heparin-Natrium	Ampoule
Isotonic NaCl solution 0,9% 10 ml	Natriumchlorid	Ampoule
Ketanest S ampoule 50 mg/2 ml	Esketamin HCl	Ampoule
Lasix ampoule 40 mg/4 ml	Furosemid	Ampoule
MCP ratio ampoule 10 mg/2 ml	Metoclopramid-HCl	Ampoule
Novaminsulfon ratio ampoule 2.5 g/5 ml	Metamizol	Ampoule
Ranitidin ratio pro injectione 50 mg/5 ml	Ranitidinhydrochlorid	Ampoule
Solu-Decortin H ampoule 250 mg	Prednisolon	Bottle
Tavegil ampoule 2 mg/5 ml	Clemastin	Ampoule

Medical Supplies/Product name	Generic name	Unit
Tramal ampoule 100 mg/2 ml	Tramadol-HCl	Ampoule
Disposable cannula, size 1		Unit
Disposable cannula, size 12		Unit
Syringe disposable 2 ml		Unit
Syringe disposable 5 ml		Unit
Syringe disposable 10 ml		Unit
Surgical disposable scalpel		Unit
Cord clamp		Unit
Antiseptic alcohol swabs		Unit
Cellulose swabs		Unit

Tab. 6   Additional medication Doctor's Kit content

Medical Supplies/Product name	Generic name	Unit
Bayotensin akut vial	Nitrendipin	Vial
Burn- and wound ointment 20 gr	Lidocain-HCl	Tube
Buscopan dragée	Butylscopolaminiumbromid	Drag.
Buscopan suppository	Butylscopolaminiumbromid	Supp.
Diazepam Desitin rectal tube 10 mg	Diazepam	Tube
Imodium Akut dragée	Loperamid-HCl	Drag.
Nitrolingual capsule	Nitroglycerin	Caps.
Paracetamol 250 suppository	Paracetamol	Supp.
Magaldrat vial	Aluminiumphosphat	Bag
Protagent eye drops	Povidon	Vial
Rectodelt suppository 100 mg	Prednison	Supp.
Vomacur dragée	Dimenhydrinat	Drag.
Vomacur 150 suppository	Dimenhydrinat	Supp.

Medical Supplies/Product name	Generic name	Unit
Documentation		
Description for use of medicine		Unit
Directions		Unit
Emergency Report		Unit
Position plan		Unit
List of content Doctor's Kit		Unit
Other (between modul suction and urinay catheder)		
Rubbish bag		Unit
Contaminated sharps container		Unit
Disposable gloves size 8.5 (non sterile)		Unit

4.2   Semi-automated external defibrillator (AED)

Every year, approximately 100,000 people in Germany succumb to sudden cardiac death, which often begins with ventricular fibrillation. The only effective countermeasure is the electrical defibrillation, which depolarizes the entire cardiac conduction system with an electrical shock. Successful application results in a normal heart rhythm. The critical factor is the early start of CPR and defibrillation, as every minute without resuscitation reduces survival rates by 10%.

Semi-automated external defibrillators (AED, see Fig. 16 and 17) have been available on board Lufthansa long-haul aircraft since the end of 1999; since

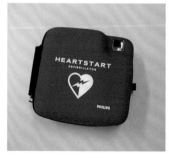

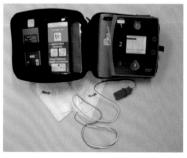

Fig. 16   AED

Fig. 17   AED (internal view)

mid-2004, short- and medium-haul aircraft have been supplied with AEDs as well.

An automated external defibrillator (AED) is a battery-powered device that displays and evaluates an ECG and provides the operator with exact directions on how to proceed. This is why these devices are easy to operate even by layrescuers.

All flight attendants are trained in the use of the AED and may apply it during the cardiopulmonary resuscitation (CPR). In this manner, the regulations of the "German Medical Devices Act" are followed, which require that only trained personnel may use an AED.

By standing medical professionals are thus relieved of the additional task of familiarizing themselves with the device, and can therefore devote their full attention to the care of the patient.

The operation of the AED is extremely simple and basically consists of turning the device on and following the verbal instructions (see Fig. 18–20).

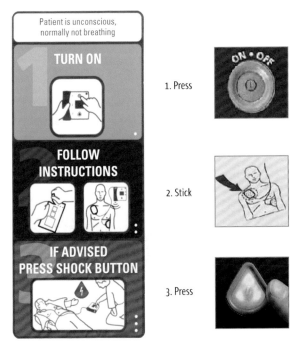

Fig. 18 Basic AED procedure

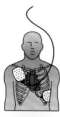

Apply the stick on
electrodes
to the exposed chest

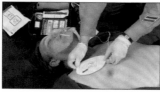

Plug in the cord
at the blinking
light

Fig. 19 AED procedure: Apply the stick on electrodes and plug in the cord

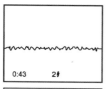

Analysis
Do not touch the patient during the analysis
Wait for device's instructions
Results of analysis:
- *Shock advised*
- *No shock advised*

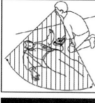

Before defibrillation
- Check if patient is not being touched
- Warnimg: *Stand clear*
- Warning: *Shocking now!*

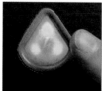

Press shock button
and follow further instructions

Fig. 20 AED procedure: Awaiting analysis and push shock button if shock is advised

It is important *not to touch the patient* during the analytical phase to avoid delays or incorrect interpretation by the device:

1. Turn on device.
2. Apply the stick-on electrodes to the exposed chest.
3. Plug in the cord at the blinking light.
4. When the verbal command "*Shock advised*" is given, press on the blinking light. At this time, do not touch the patient! Check to see that the patient is not being touched. Warn the others to "*stand clear*" and then announce "*shocking now*" before pushing the shock button.
5. Continue performing CPR until the patient regains consciousness or until emergency medical personnel can take over upon landing.

In general, the AED should *only be used on the unconscious patient during* CPR. For patients with cardiac-related complaints, the AED should be made available, but not routinely applied.

> The AED should only be used as a monitoring device in exceptional circumstances. The ECG display is not intended to be used for a definitive diagnosis and allows only limited conclusions regarding cardiac functions.

Even though there are two electrode packages included with the device, these should be saved for their "main purpose": breaking through ventricular fibrillation or pulseless ventricular tachycardia, and should not be used to casually monitor the ECG display together with the patient.

The self-adhesive electrodes, once applied, should only be removed after the patient has left the aircraft or has been handed over to emergency medical personnel. This is also the case when the patient's situation seems to have stabilized, and further measures appear to be superfluous.

4.3   Oxygen

Oxygen bottles

For the event of an *emergency*, oxygen bottles are carried along on board of the aircraft (see Fig. 21). These bottles are generally located near the flight attendant seats and may be operated by the flight attendants. They are intended primarily for the flight attendants in emergency situations, such as a rapid loss of cabin pressure, to ensure their continued mobility in the cabin to assist passengers. They are not to be used routinely for medical purposes but *only in case of an emergency*.

The on-board emergency oxygen bottles provide oxygen for over 75 minutes at a fixed flow rate of four litres per minute.

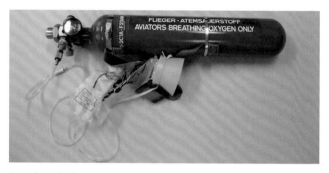

Fig. 21 Oxygen bottle

If spontaneous respiration is restored, oxygen can be provided either through the face mask (with a reservoir) or by way of nasal cannulas contained in the Doctor's Kit.

The number of bottles on board is dependent on the type of aircraft. As a general rule, one is located at every door with a flight attendant position.

Oxygen units (Wenoll WS 120 system) – additional equipment to be booked at reservation

If *continuous supplemental oxygen* is necessary, then another system is required (see Fig. 22 and 23). A carbon fibre pressure cylinder filled to 300 bars delivers, within limits, a continuous adjustable flow rate by way of an electronic regulator. The oxygen that is delivered is dependent on the inspiratory volume and the respiratory frequency through the nasal cannulas. Depending on the flow rate, *up to 14 hours of supplemental oxygen* can be achieved (see Tab. 7). The necessary setting can be predetermined by a switch. The WS 120 system can also be operated by laypeople. An instruction manual is included in the system case.

> The oxygen unit must be ordered at the time of reservation, as it is not standard equipment!

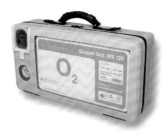

Fig. 22 Oxygen unit (external view)

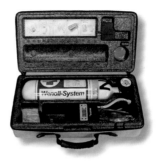

Fig. 23 Oxygen unit (internal view)

Tab. 7 Flow rate determination of the Wenoll WS 120

Selector Switch (position)	Flow Rate (l/min)	Duration of Supply (hrs)
0.5	1.2	20
0.6	2.0	16.5
0.7	2.8	14
0.8	3.6	12.5
0.9	4.4	11
1.0	5.2	10

In order to assess oxygen saturation, a *pulse oximeter* is permanently connected to the device to determine the necessary flow rate.

4.4 Satellite telephone – Medical hotline

Satellite telephones are available on long-haul aircrafts, which the flight attendants may use around the clock in the event of a medical emergency in order to obtain advices from physicians provided by a *ground medical hotline*.

In a case of emergency, flight attendants are able to connect with the ground-based medical hotline without any charges. Even though the medical incident may seem straightforward, a call to the medical hotline is recommended whenever a diversion of the flight is taken into consideration. Alongside specific emergency medical knowledge of those physicians providing medical hotline services, the fail-safe principle of four-eyes – as is usual in aviation – can thereby be counted on. Moreover, in case of diverting, the flight ground support is able to determine the best alternative airport in the nearest vicinity with regard to both medical and operational requirements.

5 Patient transport by commercial aircraft

In the early history of aviation, the advantage of transporting the ill and wounded over large distances was already evident. The year 1909 saw the first military application, using simple stretchers on single-engine airplane to transport injured soldiers. A short while later, transportation of the ill in civilian airplanes followed under similar conditions. In these early days, medical care took a sideline to the flying itself. Subsequently, especially with the development of the rescue helicopter and the PTC (Patient Transport Compartment), this relationship has completely reversed: This application has made the aircraft a resource in the provision of optimal medical care. It is hardly possible today to imagine an airline without the presence of flight attendants, who, in the end, actually hark back to a time when medical assistance was required in airplanes; the first flight attendant in aviation history was an American nurse.

The transport of patients on the ground already poses significant challenges. The condition of critically ill or injured patients can be significantly aggravated, faced with the threat of so-called "*transportation trauma*". Therefore there are two kinds of issues that must be understood. The first concerns mechanical factors such as transfer, movement and jarring, which may increase pain or lead to the dislocation of fractures. In the case of cervical vertebral fractures, incomplete immobilization can, in the worst case, lead to death. The second has to do with the strong vegetative reactions in the circulatory system, which can be difficult to control in the critically ill person, possibly leading to shock.

> Absolute requirements for the transportation of patients include:
> 1. Justifiable indication
> 2. Careful consideration of the pros and cons for the patient
> 3. Choice of the proper means of conveyance, and determination of the necessary conditions and resources

Assessing the patient's transportability and the necessary resources are physician decisions. The responsibility for the transport lies with the physician and the aviation company performing the transport. Regarding the medical care itself, the accompanying physician is in charge and takes medical responsibility for the patient. The large airline companies maintain their own medical departments which passengers, reservation agents and the airline industry may consult to obtain adequate recommendations and medical clearances. Special requirements for this activity are certification in aviation medicine and/or many years' experience with the airline.

The aforementioned basic rules should also be observed in the case of trivial medical problems. Even trifle injuries, such as ankle sprains, can lead to serious complications when associated with prolonged immobilization – for example, lethal pulmonary embolism in the absence of prophylactic anticoagulation. Questions regarding liability will, without a doubt, then be aimed at the consulting physician. Regarding air transport, the evaluation of seriously ill patients should be undertaken by an intensive care physician specialized in the appropriate medical field together with an airline physician. As a general rule, a physician who is experienced in emergency or intensive care should accompany the patient.

> Specific factors influence the decision for air transport over ground transport.

These factors can be categorized into aspects pertaining to aviation physiology, and the general conditions of flight operations.

Aviation physiology factors
1. Decrease in air pressure and partial pressure of oxygen with increasing altitude
2. Decreased humidity of the cabin air
3. Increased risk of thrombosis due to oxygen deficiency and dehydration with tendency toward oedema

4. Perspiration and increased diuresis
5. Stressors due to acceleration and movement in three-dimensional space

Unfavourable conditions of flight operations

1. Longer duration of immobilization and restricted movement
2. Limitation of therapeutic resources and interventional techniques
3. Possible conflict between optimal patient care and comfort of other passengers
4. Difficult access to clinical care in case of unforeseen deterioration of the illness

These factors should be gauged against the patient's condition, and potential complications be met by *the appropriate choice of transport type and medical resources*.

Therefore, there is a **graduated concept** which the larger airlines utilize, ranging from the simple wheelchair all the way to the fully equipped intensive care unit. After thorough consideration of the capabilities of the conveyance, the next question to answer is the necessary physical arrangement.

1. **A seated transport** can require an *additional seat*. In the case of injury, there may be the need to stretch out or elevate a leg. It should also be kept in mind that the emergency exit must not be blocked by the patient in the event of an evacuation.
2. If these measures are not adequate, the next step is to **reserve a business or first class seat**. Depending on the configuration, the seat may have a foot or leg rest available and may allow a semi-supine or a fully supine position. This option may provide the most comfortable conveyance for those with stable illnesses that do not require emergency or therapeutic interventions.
3. **Patients who must be transported supine** and require medical treatment during the flight need a so-called "stretcher" (see Fig. 24). This is a cot with fairly comfortable padding and the ability to elevate the upper body as well as to hang IV fluids. A vacuum mattress can be added to optimize fracture stabilization. In order to place such a stretcher, two rows of seats must be removed, which will raise the cost of the transport. The patient can be shielded from view of the other passengers with a curtain, allowing for privacy and provision of the proper personal care without bothering the other passengers.
4. **For critically ill patients,** especially those with existing or impending ventilator dependency, conveyance in the *Patient Transport Compartment (PTC) is obligatory*. Alternatively, an air ambulance may be required.

The PTC has so far only been used on long-haul flights of Lufthansa German Airlines AG. It provides for all types of respiratory therapies, including monitoring of blood gases and invasive cardiovascular support. Medication and equipment are similar to that found in ambulances and are within the capabilities of an intensive care unit, so that indications for transport are quite generous.

In addition to the choice of the appropriate bedding, *questions regarding boarding* must be settled (e.g. wheelchair, preboarding for stretcher), the appropriate accompaniment (relative, paramedic, nurse or physician), and the necessary medical resources (oxygen – *on demand* or *constant flow*) as well as transfer and care after the flight.

For all injured passengers with constricting dressings, immobilization and swelling as well as illnesses with elevated thrombotic potential, *antithrombotic prophylaxis* with low molecular weight heparin is highly recommended. Usually a one-time dose two hours prior to flight is adequate.

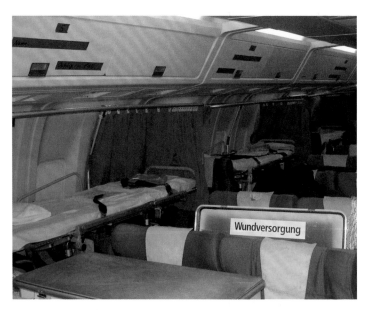

Fig. 24 Modification of Lufthansa and Condor aircraft for mass evacuation from Phuket following the tsunami in December 2004. The installation of 20 stretchers, pictured here in a Boeing 767, along with the collaboration of other airlines made it possible to rapidly repatriate about 2,500 mildly injured and 300 severely injured passengers within the first days after the disaster.

6   Intensive Care Transport

A considerable proportion of long-distance transport of patients is carried out on board of commercial airliners. This is mainly due to the more or less ubiquitous availability, the world's existing route network and lower costs per route compared e.g. to air ambulances. This holds true for intensive care transports as well. Due to the logistical and medical complexity, as far as we know only Lufthansa German Airlines provide intensive care transport capabilities for scheduled air operations on wide body aircrafts.

Lufthansa Technik AG and the Medical Service of Lufthansa AG have designed the so-called Patient Transport Compartment in the 1990s (PTC) and a modular treatment unit (Patient Transport Unit, PTU) for commercial as well as military flight operations. The PTC is to be installed in less than two hours ground time in Boeing 747-400 and Airbus A340/330 as well as A380 machines. Minor changes in aircraft design such as a so-called discharge line are required. After expanding four rows of seats an enclosed space of about 6 m² is now available (see Fig. 25).

During the flight the patient in the PTC will be accompanied by a physician of the client (usually an insurance or assistance company, as well as governmental and non-governmental organizations). Lufthansa as the responsible operator of the PTC provides an intensive care trained and experienced nurse

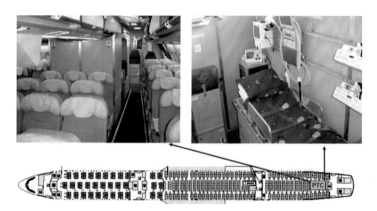

Fig. 25 PTC in Airbus A340

or paramedic (PTC Medical Crew), that is also a qualified flight attendant to guarantee both, correct handling of the patient, and devices in the PTC and emergency maneuvers whenever required.

7 Regulations regarding the transportation of ill passengers

7.1 Legal requirements

The primary mission of an airline company is to transport passengers in a timely manner according to a flight plan from one point to another. The assumption is that the passenger is well enough to tolerate the conditions of cabin altitude, dry air, oscillations, vibrations, and cramped space without difficulty. For passengers with acute illnesses on board commercial airlines, JAR OPS 1 requires that the crew of commercial aircraft is trained and current in first aid, and that the necessary on-board medical equipment is commensurate with the number of passengers. Commercial airplanes are, as a rule, not oriented toward transporting severely ill or injured passengers and patients.

Numerous requirements, such as the safety regulations pertaining to JAR OPS 1, national laws of the Federal German authorities as well as the international guidelines of the WHO and IATA, regulate the transportation of ill passengers on air carriers. The primary focus is on the safety of healthy passengers and crew, as well as the limitation of the spread of infectious diseases via world-wide flight routes.

Given the many different national and international regulations for the transportation of ill passengers on commercial airlines, it is recommended that the affected passenger, whether acutely or chronically ill, notifies the airline prior to boarding in order to avoid complications.

In general, most airlines align their policies according to IATA's recommendations for ill and disabled passengers.

7.2   General guidelines for medical clearance of ill passengers

These general guidelines refer to passengers with acute or unstable medical conditions.

It is illegal to transport infectious passengers in commercial aircraft!

The following passengers are basically deemed not fit to fly and **require medical clearance by the medical department** of the airline company or a flight surgeon respectively:

- All cases of *communicable disease,* or diseases that can be transmitted by the passenger
- Passengers with *physical or mental disabilities* that can endanger the operation of the flight or can significantly restrict the comfort of other passengers
- When the condition of the passenger puts the *safety of the flight at risk* or may provoke an unplanned intermediate landing
- Passengers who *cannot take care of themselves* and require special support
- Passengers whose medical condition can *deteriorate significantly* due to the physiological demands of the flight

Passengers who do not fall into any of these categories are generally fit to fly.

If any doubt exists, medical consultation with the respective airline should be sought in every case.

7.3   Medical clearance – General rules of Lufthansa

Patients will be **excluded from commercial flights if they:**

- Are a danger to themselves or others, despite specific precautionary measures during the flight
- Based on their physical or mental condition, are not in the position to care for themselves during the flight, but want to travel without adequate escort

- Represent a source of infection
- Are unable to use the regular aircraft seats in an upright or reclined position

A medical evaluation prior to flight either by the medical department of Lufthansa or one of its authorized contract physicians in foreign stations is required when:

- The passenger is considered contagious with a communicable disease
- The passenger's physical or mental state may lead to a hazardous situation
- The passenger constitutes a potential health risk
- The passenger is not able to care for him- or herself
- The medical condition of the passenger is likely to deteriorate during, or because of, the flight

For Lufthansa, **approval for flight** by the medical department or a contract physician is generally required for passengers with:

- Significant external injuries after medical treatment
- Internal injuries
- Brain lesions or skull injuries
- Hemi- or tetraplegia

8 Legal aspects of medical assistance on board commercial aircraft

8.1 Decision-making authority on board

The provision of medical assistance on the ground can involve a variety of legal issues, especially when the outcome is not as desired. This is equally true for assistance provided in the air. Here, however, the situation is further complicated by the fact that the medical volunteer provides such assistance in an unfamiliar environment using unfamiliar medical equipment, often under significantly more difficult conditions. While a doctor may be "king of the castle" in his or her own clinical practice or hospital, this is by no means the case in the air: Decision-making on board can give rise to conflicts when the judgement of the doctor differs from that of the captain. A conceivable example would be a situation in which a doctor is called to assist a passenger on board and decides that the ill passenger needs immediate admission to a hospital. Unfortunately, however, this decision is reached precisely when the aircraft is flying over Greenland, where a severe snowstorm is raging, or over Saudi Arabia, where an unexpected sandstorm makes an intermediate landing very dangerous. Despite the pleadings of the doctor to make an unscheduled landing, the captain decides against it, and the passenger dies.

Who is ultimately responsible for the decision to make an unscheduled landing?

Section 3 of the German Aviation Regulation *(Luftverkehrs-Ordnung, LuftVO)* specifies that the captain has decision-making authority over the aircraft (so-called nautical authority). Section 12 of the newly introduced German Aviation Security Act *(Luftsicherheitsgesetz, LuftSiG)* specifies that the captain is responsible for maintaining safety and order on board the aircraft.

> It hence follows that the captain alone decides whether it is possible to comply with a doctor's recommendation to perform an unscheduled landing.

According to the abovementioned Aviation Security Act, *the ultimate decision lies with the captain*. The moral, ethical and legal obligation of the doctor to provide first aid reaches its limits where the authority of the captain begins: All persons on board are required to follow the instructions of the captain (Section 12 subsection 2 of the Aviation Security Act).

It must, however, be pointed out that this allocation of decision-making authority only results in differences of opinion in exceptional cases. In general, the captain is relieved and thankful when a medically trained person actually responds and offers assistance when a distressed flight attendant calls out "Is there a doctor on board?".

Increasingly often this question is heard at cruising altitudes – and usually successfully elicits a response, as, *on average, three out of four times there actually is a doctor or another medically trained person on board*. Not only the ill passenger, but the airline, too, depends on the assistance of this volunteer, as no legal regulations whatsoever require airlines to provide emergency medical assistance or medically trained personnel on board their aircraft. An airline is obligated to provide transportation from point A to point B, and is required to do so in a technically safe manner. It is not obligated to provide on-board medical care for ill passengers by airline personnel. However, it does have the obligation to attempt to locate a medically trained individual on board and to afford that individual the best conceivable means for providing such care under the circumstances. These "best conceivable means" include appropriate emergency medical equipment on board the aircraft. The regulatory agencies of most countries have set out minimum recommendations for such equipment. However, there are significant differences from country to country. Not the least for this reason, EASA, the European Aviation Safety Agency, has issued rules to ensure that the medical equipment on board of the aircraft is not only standardized but also uniformly complete and comprehensive. A uniform standard is also applied concerning the extent to which crew members can be called upon to operate on-board medical equipment such as defibrillators.

8.2 Failure to render assistance on board also punishable by law

A doctor who for ethical reasons unhesitatingly responds to a flight attendant's request for assistance may later face uncomfortable consequences for having rendered this assistance – including potential legal consequences.

If, for example, the volunteer doctor after enjoying several glasses of strong red wine with dinner or for other reasons, has committed a medical error while rendering assistance in an unfamiliar environment or even with inadequate equipment, it is possible that the patient – or, in the case of death, his or her survivors – will sue the doctor for malpractice. Would it not therefore be more prudent for the doctor to pretend not to have heard the desperate flight attendant's call for medical assistance – perhaps by feigning sleep? Not necessarily, as there are many countries, among them France and Australia, that have laws similar to Section 323c of the German Criminal Code (*Strafgesetzbuch, StGB*), which reads:

> **Section 323c, German Criminal Code**: Whoever does not render assistance during accidents
> … although it is required and can be expected of him or her under the circumstances
> … shall be punished with imprisonment for not more than one year or a fine.

And French, Australian or German law might not only be applicable as long as the aircraft in which the first aid is provided is in the airspace over French, Australian or German territory. Indeed, one of the principles of international law, and thus also of aviation law, – "*cuius solum, eius coelum*" – applies, meaning that the national law of a state is applicable within its territory and adjacent waters as well as in the airspace above its territory and adjacent waters. Often, however, states are not in a position to apply or enforce their laws and regulations within their airspace. Consider the hijacking of an airplane: Which national criminal law shall apply when the errant aircraft flies over several countries? Often these countries do not even have an interest in applying their laws, at least in the case of an overflight – the situation may be different in the case of a landing.

Over time, therefore, territorial law has increasingly given way to the law of the flag: The law of the flag applies to all activity – or inactivity – on board an aircraft, irrespective of the aircraft's location. Failure to render medical assistance on board an aircraft cruising through the airspace of a foreign country can thus be judged according to the national law of the aircraft's flag state. On-board treatment of an ill passenger is subject to the same national law as well. If the person rendering assistance makes a medical error, he or she may find him- or herself faced with criminal proceedings initiated by an overzealous prosecutor or civil proceedings initiated by the passenger or his or her survivors – or both types of proceedings simultaneously. Similarly, the national criminal law of the respective state may also apply in the case of failure to render assistance even though such assistance was called for and could reasonably have been expected.

8.3 Liability insurance coverage for the provision of first aid on board

Such potential legal consequences do not necessarily encourage the provision of first aid. For this reason, Lufthansa German Airlines AG and its affiliated companies as well as numerous other airlines offer liability insurance coverage for doctors and other persons rendering assistance. Under the corresponding provisions of the Lufthansa insurance policy ("Medical Assistance on Board"), for instance, liability insurance coverage is provided for doctors and other persons rendering assistance on board the aircraft of the companies insured under the policy. Excluded, however, are damages caused by their wilful intent.

> *Whosoever provides first aid on board an aircraft belonging to the Lufthansa Group, whether a doctor or other person rendering assistance, shall enjoy liability insurance coverage against all claims that the passenger, his or her survivors, or his or her social insurance carrier may make.*

The medical volunteer is even deemed to be a co-insured, i.e. Lufthansa's insurer places him or her on the same footing as its insured, Lufthansa, and will take over litigation and assume the associated costs as well as any compensation payments the medical volunteer may be sentenced to make. Within the framework of this extensive indemnity, the assertion of a right of recourse against the medical volunteer is also waived, even if damages were caused by that person's gross negligence.

> **No insurance clause without an exception**
> There is no indemnity and no assumption of liability in the event that the medical volunteer wilfully causes harm – admittedly an extremely unlikely scenario.

With the inclusion of this extensive assumption of liability in its insurance policy, Lufthansa takes on the financial risk of medical volunteerism. While the volunteer's medical malpractice insurance could in principle be utilized as well, as it makes no difference whether assistance is provided on the ground or in the air, it is questionable whether every malpractice policy would also provide coverage abroad or cover medical errors attributable to gross negligence. Through the coverage provided under the Lufthansa liability insurance policy, the volunteer's medical malpractice insurance would in any case remain unblemished.

Very few airlines offer indemnity as comprehensive as that provided by Lufthansa. In some cases special exclusions are agreed, such as no indemnity for malpractice claims lodged in the United States or Canada. The reason for this exclusion is the sometimes exorbitant compensation awarded to plaintiffs by courts in those countries. In the last few years, however, the situation has improved in the United States in that all the constituent states have enacted so-called "Good Samaritan" legislation. (For those who would like to read the story of the Good Samaritan: Luke 10:30–37). Under such legislation the individual who voluntarily performs "Good Samaritan" acts in the event of an emergency is indemnified against all liability claims unless he or she causes bodily injury through gross negligence. The expectation of financial compensation for such assistance, however, removes the element of voluntariness. This more recent American legislation has thus mitigated the exclusions in some malpractice policies, at least for the United States.

8.4 Liability of medical volunteers under criminal law

Lufthansa's insurance policy cannot – for understandable reasons – cover potential prosecution of medical volunteers under criminal law. Criminal consequences can arise, *inter alia*, if a doctor makes a *medical error* while providing assistance on board. According to the jurisprudence of the courts in Germany, medical intervention *per se* is deemed to constitute bodily injury. This applies even to those medical interventions which were performed for therapeutic purposes with the requisite professional skill and were successful. According to the courts, however, the intervention itself – and hence the bodily injury – is deemed to be justified by the express or implied *informed consent of the patient*. In the absence of such consent, the intervention can be justified on grounds of agency without specific authorization or by a legitimate emergency. This is the case, for example, when an intervention must be performed immediately on a non-communicative or unconscious patient. Therefore, if the doctor recognizes that an unconscious patient is a member of a religious community that does not allow certain medical interventions on religious grounds, the intervention should not be performed until informed consent can be obtained. If the doctor negligently fails to recognize that informed consent has not been given, or negligently believes that consent has been given, then punishment pursuant to the criminal provisions on negligent bodily injury would indeed be conceivable.

With regard to possible criminal liability of doctors for their conduct, the regime applicable in the air is essentially not different from the regime applicable on the ground. However, there are additional *defences* that can assist the volunteer doctor in the air: He or she may have rendered assistance in an unfamiliar environment, he or she may have been dealing with a patient with whom it was impossible to communicate due to language difficulties, or the volunteer doctor may have been faced with an emergency situation where swift action was necessary. These extenuating circumstances should make it extremely hard for a public prosecutor to charge a doctor or other person rendering assistance with negligent bodily injury.

The requirements set out by the courts in respect of the *doctor's duty to take care* and *duty to inform* in order to avoid fulfilling the elements constituting bodily injury make it more burdensome for doctors to meet all of these requirements. On the other hand, the courts appear to be finding it increasingly difficult to assess the factual and economic consequences of the requirements they impose on doctors and hospital operators. The challenge to the courts must therefore be to not lose touch with reality and, in the interests of both patients and doctors, clearly distinguish between what is desirable and what is economically feasible.

8.5   Honorarium for doctors

The claim is often raised, especially by doctors' associations in the United States and Great Britain, that airlines should pay an appropriate honorarium to persons rendering medical assistance. Individual doctors have already gone to court in an attempt to claim payment of a honorarium for assistance rendered during a flight.

> In principle, such a claim to an honorarium from an airline is not justifiable!

When an airline requests the assistance of a doctor on board, it is not doing so to safeguard its own interests but instead to safeguard the interests of the ill passenger. To be sure, the airline is responsible for the safe transportation of the passenger from the airport of departure to the airport of destination, but its duty to take care applies only in regard to the technically safe performance of the flight. Damage to the health of passengers which is not connected to the technically safe performance of the flight, i.e. damage originating in the physical condition of the passenger, does not fall within the airline's scope of responsibility. Contrary to popular opinion, an airline is not its passengers' life insurance company!

> When a doctor's assistance is requested on board, the airline is taking this action by authorization of the passenger or, if the passenger is no longer in a position to give such authorization, by agency of necessity without specific authorization but in the interest of the passenger. When examining and treating the passenger, the

doctor is thus not acting primarily in the interest of the airline, although it is also in the airline's interest to continue the flight without further disruption. He or she is acting primarily in the interest of and on behalf of the passenger.

Any claims for payment of an honorarium, insofar as they are to be made at all, would in any case have to be addressed to the passenger, with all the difficulties this could entail for the doctor. The situation would be a different one only if the airline, through negligent actions of its employees, caused bodily injury to a passenger. If, for example, a flight attendant pours boiling hot coffee into a passenger's lap instead of his or her cup, the hailed doctor is acting in the interest of the airline, and an honorarium could then more likely be considered appropriate than in a case in which the doctor is acting only on behalf of the passenger.

As stated before, under the American "Good Samaritan" legislation the medical volunteer is largely relieved of liability for negligence. The prerequisite, however, is that the assistance be provided voluntarily. One can no longer speak of voluntariness, however, if the assistance is followed up by a demand for payment of an honorarium. In one such case, American courts denied indemnity against claims under civil law, holding that in the provision of the assistance that was ethically called for in the case at hand, financial considerations had outweighed the element of voluntariness.

> A doctor's claims to an honorarium from an airline were recently dismissed by a British court. On a flight from Los Angeles to London, a British doctor had provided first aid to a passenger who had suffered a blood clot. His request for payment of 540 GBP was refused by airline A.A., and his legal action was also unsuccessful in court. The passenger found this unbelievable: "I am astonished by the behaviour of A.A. The doctor saved my life, I could have died – why doesn't A. A. pay him?" The passenger's words quoted in the newspaper "The Irish Independent" reflect a total misunderstanding of the duties incumbent upon the passenger as a patient.

8.6 Transmission of infectious diseases through aircraft

The respiratory disease SARS lies behind us – and avian the next period of influenza possibly lies ahead.

> SARS caused greater economic losses for international aviation than the events of September 11 and the first Iraq war combined.

Millions of air travellers avoided flights within or to Asia. The same thing can occur again if avian influenza actually breaks out extensively. In the event of an outbreak of such an epidemic, even a liability of the airlines cannot be excluded: namely, if they culpably violate precautionary measures stipulated in pertinent legislation and such violation is the cause of infection of passengers or even third parties.

In Germany, the legal basis for action against airlines in such cases is the *Protection Against Infection Act (Infektionsschutzgesetz, IfSG)*. It specifies very detailed obligations of the local public health authorities, such as the obligation to exclude infected persons from air transport, the obligation to protect aircraft on the ground in areas where there are outbreaks of infectious diseases, and the obligation to perform disinfection procedures. In addition, IATA Regulation 700 provides for a right of the airlines to exclude infected persons from air transport.

Violation by the airlines of the provisions of the Protection Against Infection Act is quite conceivable: e.g. failure to refuse to transport a passenger despite suspicion of illness, failure to *isolate suspected ill passengers* during a flight, failure to subsequently *notify other passengers* after an ill passenger has been identified, or failure to inform public health authorities about such an event. If one of these omissions could have been responsible for the spread of a disease, the question of a liability of the airline is quickly raised – but less eaily answered.

Infected passengers can also make claims against airlines on the basis of the so-called *Montreal Convention*. The prerequisite for liability under this Convention is that an "accident" must have occurred. Here, however, the term "accident" does not mean a (traffic) accident in the commonly understood sense of the word. Rather, an "accident" within the meaning of the Montreal Convention is a sudden event or occurrence that is external to the passenger and has a negative impact on his or her health. An illness, lacking the element of suddenness, is not likely to fulfil the criteria of such an "accident". Additionally, an illness usually does not break out on board, but rather later, so that the question arises whether placing the cause on board is still sufficient for establishing such liability if the ensuing risk did not materialize until after the end of the relevant period of liability, namely after the conclusion of carriage by air. However, it is entirely conceivable that ancillary obligations arising from the contract of carriage may have been breached, such as the obligation in the event of an identified risk of infection to warn all passengers who may have come into contact with the infected passenger.

> During the SARS crisis, for instance, Lufthansa had to warn passengers on a flight from Hong Kong to Frankfurt who had travelled in the same compartment as the infected person. Moreover, because this passenger subsequently flew to Spain, all the other passengers on the subsequent flight also had to be informed of their possible risk of infec-

tion. Fulfilment of this duty to warn was only possible with the assistance of the local public health authorities and the media. Further complicating fulfilment of the duty to warn is the fact that not only in Germany but also in many other countries, strict data protection laws are in force which make it considerably more difficult for airlines or the authorities to obtain contact information.

8.7   The (growing) role of doctors in aviation litigation

The role of the medical community in aviation will probably continue to grow in the future, as passengers or their lawyers will increasingly be calling medical experts into the courtroom to testify in passenger liability litigation. The reason behind this is that in the last few years there have been profound changes in the liability regime of aviation law. Previously, in cases of death or bodily injury of passengers, the liability of airlines was limited financially. This liability limit could only be broken if the injured party was able to prove wilful misconduct or gross negligence on the part of the airline – which was nearly impossible to prove. The lawyers' art at the time was to try to furnish such proof and thus obtain more than just limited liability compensation for their clients.

Meanwhile, the liability regime has been changed: Now the liability of the airline is no longer limited, but unlimited up to the amount of the proven damages. The focus of the lawyers' argumentation and submission of evidence has consequently shifted from an attempt to break the liability limit to an attempt to construct and prove the highest possible personal injury damages.

The law awards *compensation for damages in the event of death or bodily injury* of the passenger. And this apparently clear regulation is where the difficulties begin: There is, in fact, considerable dispute as to whether this regulation encompasses psychological damages in addition to physical damages. It is precisely psychological damages such as emotional shock, trauma, and anxiety that can hardly be refuted by the defendant, i.e. the airline. If, after a flight through bad weather or a hard landing, a passenger claims to suffer from fear of flying, can the airline prove otherwise? Especially in the United States, the passengers – or, as the case may be, their attorneys – have availed themselves of the services of the medical community in order to expound and attempt to prove the most far-fetched theories of anxiety. The courts have quickly put a stop to such endeavours, however, holding that psychological damages by themselves, in other words, isolated from and independent of physical damages, are not compensable. This makes sense, as only those who have suffered physical damages may be believed to have suffered psychological damages as well.

Some claimants, however, have managed to surmount this barrier erected by the courts: The court of appeals in Montana (USA), for instance, namely held that "post-traumatic stress disorder" (PTSD) claimed by a passenger as a consequence of evacuation from an aircraft could be considered bodily injury, i.e. physical damages. The attending doctor had proven in court – at least the court believed him – that the consequences of the evacuation had triggered biochemical reactions in the passenger's body that in turn affected the passenger's brain and neurological system. This, he said, represented a classic case of PTSD, and PTSD arose from changes in "brain chemistry", physiology, and anatomy. The claimant had therefore suffered a brain injury, the doctor continued, because allegedly – according to recent scientific studies – PTSD represented trauma to the cellular structure of the brain. Fear alone, the court held, did not qualify for compensation, but a brain injury that had its origin in fear did. One can only ungrudgingly acknowledge that the doctor providing this expert opinion did a good job. But then how many brain cells must have been destroyed in soldiers who saw combat in wars and really experienced fear?!

Another similarly bizarre stance taken by American courts is the awarding of compensation for *"pre-impact conscious pain and suffering"*. In the United States, compensation for such pain and suffering is awarded not only to passengers – if they survive an accident – but also to their survivors in two different types of situations:

- In the first type of situation, the passenger is aware for an extended period of time that the airplane will crash. The classic case is the passenger of an A.A. DC-10 who allegedly saw an engine fall off the wing after take-off from Chicago and allegedly knew that his aircraft was immediately going to crash. It is questionable, however, whether the passenger actually saw the engine fall off or whether he was reading his newspaper. Nonetheless, the court awarded the survivors compensation for pain and suffering.
- The second type of situation arises when in all probability it can be assumed that the passenger survived the accident itself – if only for a brief time – and recognized that this accident would have serious, and perhaps even fatal consequences for him or her. This conclusion cannot be drawn without the assistance of doctors. The doctor must at least attempt to prove that the passenger in question initially survived the accident, feared for his or her life, suffered pain, and then later died. As a rule, however, such "proof" is likely to be based largely on speculation and to border on charlatanry. Here the art of medicine is misused by lawyers in order to achieve a dubious goal: Can I really say with sufficient certainty whether and how long a passenger survived and consciously experienced an accident? And can such a determination be taken as grounds for compensation for pain and suffering that is awarded not to the passenger but to his or her survivors?

Up until fairly recently, under German aviation law – contrary to the situation under other legal systems – only material damages such as the costs associated with medical care, loss of income, maintenance claims or burial expenses were reimbursable. Since 1 August 2002, however, immaterial damages such as pain and suffering have also been compensable. One can only hope that in the course of compensating immaterial damages the German legal system will not go the way of the American legal system. When "big money" is concerned, however, German lawyers unfortunately learn very quickly – as do some doctors. The object here is not to deny passengers reasonable compensation to which they are entitled. It is instead to prevent collusion between lawyers and doctors with the sole aim of artificially exaggerating medical problems or injuries.

8.8   The so-called "economy class syndrome"

Commercial aviation has existed for nearly 100 years. Only in the last few years, however, has one heard and read about a phenomenon that apparently did not exist in earlier times: thrombosis as a result of long flights, also referred to by the scientifically incorrect term "economy class syndrome". Doctors know that this disorder can develop from lengthy sitting elsewhere as well. What is surprising is that after the first claim was lodged in Australia, similar claims were also lodged in numerous other countries. At least in England and Australia, even class actions were initiated, i.e. lawsuits collectively brought by numerous allegedly affected individuals against various airlines. Among the claimants were several passengers who had allegedly developed thromboses after flights lasting merely two or three hours. A point of attack had finally been found against the airlines: Though aware of the risk of thrombosis, it was asserted, the airlines forced their passengers into narrow seat rows, hindered them from getting up and leaving their seats during the flight and additionally neglected to issue warnings regarding the alleged relationship between seat pitch and risk of thrombosis.

The first lawsuits have been lodged in Germany as well. One claim was dismissed with final and binding effect; in another action the court of first instance ruled against the plaintiff. A third claim was settled, albeit on other grounds, whereby the plaintiff accepted a settlement of less than 2% of the amount originally claimed in the lawsuit – a settlement that did not even cover her court costs.

Particularly noteworthy is the lawsuit first decided by the Frankfurt Regional Court and subsequently upheld by the Frankfurt Higher Regional Court. The defendant claimed to have developed a pulmonary embolism as a result of a thrombosis contracted on a flight in economy class from Frankfurt to

Johannesburg. He did not seek medical care in Johannesburg upon arrival, however, but instead continued on a safari. He allegedly also developed a pulmonary embolism on the return flight 10 days later. Upon returning to Germany, he finally sought medical care. The Frankfurt Regional Court found no breach of duty by the airline and dismissed the defendant's claim on essentially the following grounds:

> Not least due to widespread media attention for court decisions in the USA dealing with product liability, the attitude that there is no longer a general risk associated with daily life has also become increasingly prevalent in Germany. This attitude fails to recognize the fact that our environment has become exceedingly dangerous as a result of a multitude of discoveries and inventions in the fields of chemistry and technology. Every citizen who is competent to handle his or her own affairs, reads the newspaper, watches television and attentively observes his or her environment is aware of these dangers. Chemistry in the form of medicines, for instance, as well as technology of all kinds offer undreamed-of comforts and conveniences in everyday life and in some cases serve to prolong life, but only if one keeps an eye out for and avoids the dangers inevitably inherent in them.

> The product liability laws in force today merely obligate the given manufacturer to refrain from creating any extraordinary dangers and to point out perils that the normally responsible consumer cannot be expected to discern even if he or she exercises due care. Under no circumstances can product manufacturers be expected to relieve users of every risk associated with everyday living, essentially equating them with people who are incompetent to handle their own affairs. These are the standards by which the due diligence of the airline in this case must be judged.

> Furthermore, the defendant airline offers an exercise programme via an in-flight video that is shown on every long-haul flight. The company also funded an extensive and expensive study on the thrombosis problem and supported a corresponding dissertation. The outcome of the study and the dissertation was that the risk of thrombosis on long-haul flights is no greater than in the case of any other sedentary activity. Therefore the airline did not create any increased danger that would have necessitated a heightened level of due diligence.

With these refreshingly clear and welcome words, the Frankfurt Regional Court put a stop to the claimant's attempt to shift the general risk associated with everyday living – insofar as it had even manifested itself – onto the airline. The Frankfurt Higher Regional Court upheld the decision of the Regional Court. The decision is now final and binding. In the meantime, a second lawsuit has been dismissed by the Frankfurt Higher Regional Court with final and binding effect.

In other countries, too, the overwhelming majority of lawsuits have been decided in favour of the airlines. The courts rightly referred to a lack of proof of causality or to a general risk associated with everyday living that must simply be taken as given, so there is good reason to hope that such lawsuits will no longer arise.

II

Preflight advice

1 Medications, checklists, travel medicine

Every trip ultimately represents a physically as well as psychosocially stressful situation. With proactive planning and consideration of the characteristics of an airline trip, such as night flight, time zones changes, different climates, etc., many of these difficulties can be prevented.

Approximately six to eight weeks in advance, a *health examination* should be carried out by a general practitioner. Vaccination status should be verified with regard to the destination, updated, and additionally required immunization provided. Likewise, a *dental examination* and cleaning should be performed, especially when chronic inflammation exists.

In cases of *chronic illness*, an adequate *supply of medications* should be obtained. These should be packed into the carry-on luggage, in the event that the checked luggage is delayed upon arrival. Additionally, the *certificate of health/ medical report* regarding the medical condition(s) should be written in English, and (ideally!) also in the language of the destination country. Likewise, the names and addresses of local doctors and clinics should be provided, as the hotel or resort doctors are not always the best solution. The tourist bureau or travel agency can be helpful in this regard.

If medications are taken regularly, especially when timing of dosage is critical (such as with insulin-dependent diabetes mellitus, glaucoma, severe hypertension, anti-coagulation, etc.), one must consider time-zone changes in order to adjust adminis-tration smoothly to the new local time.

Furthermore, it must be taken into consideration that many medications have different effects in relationship to the time of ingestion (chronophar-macological effects). Time zone tables or electronic travel information for-mats are helpful in making such adjustments.

1.1 Preflight checklists

Before embarking on a trip, it is worth to list important points concerning medical issues in the form of a checklist, to proofread it and keep it in a se-cure place. This ensures that neither travel immunizations nor routine med-ications will be forgotten.

A particularly important additional point is that the *security regulations in aviation* are becoming increasingly strict, and vary from country to country.

For example, medications in carry-on luggage may only be in the amount required for one day, and must be accompanied by a certificate from the physician docu-menting its necessity!

As a variety of issues, such as vaccinations and certifications, should be taken care of in the weeks prior to travel, it is reasonable to keep a calendar in order to keep track of the respective deadlines. In addition to the health-related concerns, applications for visas and the expiration dates of personal documents should also be taken into consideration.

1.1.1 Personal documents

Many countries require a minimum period of validity for passports or other types of official identification – as a rule, usually at least six months from the time of departure. Applications for the required visas must be made in time, with attention paid to the expiration dates, so that the visa does not expire during the stay, in the event that the trip is delayed.

For children under 12 years of age, a children's passport or appropriate entry in the passport of a parent is sufficient in many countries. However, some countries require a regular passport for children regardless of age, the same as is issued to adults. Questions regarding such requirements should be directed to the embassy or consulate of the respective country!

With regard to the duration of stay and the reason for the visit, a variety of countries require an official *medical certification of a negative HIV test* which also must be issued within a specified period of time prior to entry. This is generally only required for long-term stays for business purposes. Furthermore, one should check whether other health declarations are required as well. Apart from the different travel medicine information media, the information provided by the official representatives of the countries in question should be followed.

> **Personal documents**
> - Take note of expiration dates!
> - Is a visa required?
> - Entry requirements regarding health declarations, such as immunizations or HIV tests!

1.1.2 General precautions: Medical check-up! Immunizations! Dentist!

Particularly when preparing for a lengthy stay, but even for shorter vacations, e.g. in tropical regions, a *preventive health examination* is recommended. In addition to individual consultation regarding chronic medical conditions, this process will also result in a review of vaccination status. However, not all types of travel immunizations are covered by health insurers.

> **Routine immunizations:** Tetanus, diphtheria, poliomyelitis, pertussis, measles, mumps, rubella, varicella, (possibly hepatitis A)
>
> **Travel immunizations:** Yellow fever, typhus, rabies, hepatitis B (cholera, if necessary)

Particular attention should be paid regarding *yellow fever immunization*. It is only recognized if administered by an officially certified agency and documented with the proper stamp. Stamps or certificates from general practitioners or hospitals are not accepted. Yellow fever immunization is performed by specifically licensed physicians, or by institutes or hospitals for tropical medicine, port physicians or public health agencies.

Apart from immunizations, one should also seek recommendations for prophylaxis against *tropical diseases* such as *malaria, dengue fever, and schistosomiases* in a timely manner. An additional consideration is personal protective equipment, such as the choice of clothing and insect repellent, as well as personal hygiene rules. One should also give *chemoprophylaxis* some thought.

In addition to the personal medical examination, one should not forget a visit to the *dentist*. While medical care at holiday destinations is largely acceptable, the same cannot be said for dental care. In acute cases, the dental philosophy is not always that of tooth preservation, but rather of dental extraction!

1.1.3 Documentation

The traveller should carry documentation (in English, as well as in the local language if possible) regarding his or her *chronic illnesses*. This significantly simplifies medical treatment in foreign countries. A health insurance certificate that is valid in other European countries is necessary, or, when travelling outside of Europe, an international health insurance policy which includes repatriation.

In the wake of the steady increase of anti-terrorism security measures on airplanes, *medical equipment such as insulin pens and syringes* may only be brought on board if official medical documentation (in English) is presented.

Equipment such as inhalation devices or nebulizers, oxygen equipment, and other devices may only be used on board if previously *approved by the respective airline and the national aviation agency*. This being the case for limited number of equipment types, these should be packed with the checked luggage and not brought on board in carry-on bags.

> Documentation (multiple languages) for:
> - Chronic medical conditions and medications
> - Medical equipment, such as insulin pens, inhalation devices, nebulizers, or blood glucometers (if use on board is necessary)

1.2 Personal travel medications

Travel medications are made up of two parts:

1. The weekly supply of *medications that are needed daily* (such as antihypertensives, cardiac or diabetic medications) belongs in the hand luggage (with documentation!). Additional supplies can be packed in the checked luggage.
2. The assortment of *required medication (travel medicines)*, which will be stowed in checked luggage, is determined by the destination.

The following accidents and medical problems should be provided for:

- Minor injuries
- Sprains and strains
- Bronchial infections, cough
- Motion sickness
- Traveller's diarrhoea
- Insect stings and bites
- Allergic reactions (local and systemic therapies)
- Non-specific fevers
- Gastrointestinal cramps
- Non-specific pain
- Gall bladder and renal colic
- Rheumatic complaints

Recommendations for specific preparations or drug classes will not be made here. There are far too many, and every person has individual experiences regarding the effectiveness of medications and can therefore make his or her own choices.

2   Time zone changes

Many bodily functions are influenced by circadian rhythms. They are governed by a variety of control functions. First and foremost is daylight, which regulates waking and sleeping, but also hunger and thirst. Equally important for the regulation of important body functions is the release of a variety of hormones, such as from the adrenal or hypophyseal gland, which fluctuates over the course of the day. Sleep is influenced by the daily secretion of melatonin. Other examples are blood pressure, blood sugar, or body temperature. Other non-symptomatic consequences are the levels of electrolytes or catecholamines. Even a variety of different illnesses, such as myocardial infarction, which is more likely to occur in the early morning hours, follow a daily rhythm. Less well known is that medications have a variable effect depending on time of ingestion, a phenomenon called chronopharmocology.

If the body is exposed to another *time zone* (see Fig. 26), it requires a certain period of time to adjust to the disturbed rhythms, which are determined primarily by daylight.

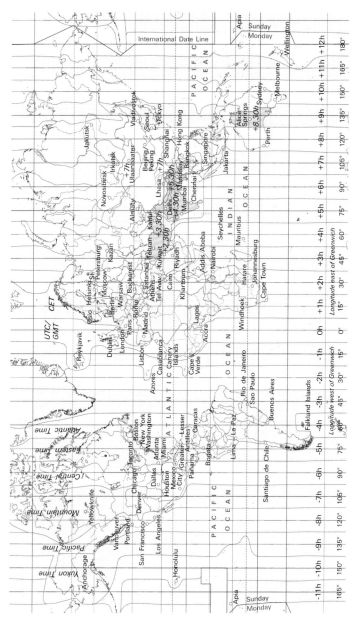

Fig. 26 Time zones

> Experience has shown that, generally, every hour of time zone difference requires an adjustment period of 24 hours.

A voyage by ship from Europe to the east coast of the United States takes about six days, with a time zone shift of minus six hours; therefore the clock is set back every day by one hour and no one notices any problems with this westward time zone shift.

The familiar and noticeable effect of *jet lag* arose with modern aviation, and particularly with the development of jet airliners. Because of their high speeds, many time zones can be crossed in a few hours. For example, a morning flight departing from Europe can reach New York in about seven hours, while the local time there is only one hour later than that of departure. This inevitably leads to a desynchronization of the circadian rhythm, including the deregulation of glandular secretions in their proper sequences. Sleep/wake cycles, temperature and blood pressure and vegetative functions such as hunger and thirst, or gastrointestinal functions, are disturbed. This *desynchronization* is not to be viewed as an illness, but rather as being in the realm of subjective sensation disturbances, even if performance is objectively decreased until complete adaptation to the new time zones is established.

Forward time zone changes are tolerated better!

Experience has shown that westward flights which lengthen the day are tolerated better than flights toward the east which shorten the day. The latter is felt to be significantly more uncomfortable, and requires more time for resynchronization. For each time zone change of one hour, in general (e.g. vacation) a period of 24 hours is adequate, albeit not optimal. However, at least three to five days per hour of time zone change are needed to establish the usual performance abilities (e.g. athletes travelling to world competitions). Slight shifts of various cycles, such as catecholamine levels, can be detected even after three weeks.

Therefore, the following recommendations for different kinds of travellers are provided:

- The business traveller, usually overseas for short periods of time, should stay within his or her home time zone to the extent possible, as far as appointments and deadlines allow.
- Vacation travellers, on the other hand, naturally want to adjust swiftly to local time zones. During the flight, they can take a two- to three-hour nap, or at least insert a rest period. On arrival at the destination,

after travelling in a westerly direction and thus lengthening the day, they should immediately jump into the schedule of the local time zone. This means that despite being fatigued by the flight, they should have a light evening meal and go to bed at about 10 p.m. In this manner, they will experience light sleep disturbances the first two or three nights, but overcome the westward shift quickly.

Eastward flights are more problematic!

Eastbound flights generally leave in the early or even late evening hours. Here it is reasonable, following on-board service, to disregard the movie, music, and the like, and to try to get as much sleep as possible. Again, the diurnal cycles of body temperature and blood pressure with their characteristic morning lows come to bear. This easily leads to a feeling of cold and disturbed sleep. Wearing warm clothes can help. Since arrival usually is in the late morning, a shortened night with suboptimal sleep has passed, yet one can arrive relatively fresh and directly adopt the local time. Subsequent nights will most likely be characterized by light sleep disturbances.

To shorten or avoid jet lag?

Melatonin is often mentioned in this regard. With its day-and-night rhythm, this hormone is an essential sleep regulator. Studies have shown a significant positive effect. Time zone changes of 12 hours can be resynchronized in half the usual time with use of melatonin. An eight-hour time zone shift is still reduced by 20%, although there seems to be no proven effect with a six-hour time zone difference. In these studies melatonin was substituted in doses of 100 mg/d, and even 1000 mg/d in Australian studies. There are no confirmed findings as to the dosage of substitution, and even less is known about side effects, especially when used long-term.

> The recommendation to adapt to the new time zone while still in the home time zone by shifting sleep/wake cycles is rather impractical, considering the period of time that is available for vacation.

Practical recommendations for inflight behaviour

Cabin service can be enjoyed without worries. The physiology of nutrition is such that a carbohydrate meal induces sleep. Protein-rich foods, such as steak, have hindering effects. This should also be kept in mind for the first few days after arrival. Alcohol consumption is also discouraged, with the following recommendation: Alcohol-induced sleep has a variety of negative effects, such as gastrointestinal immobility, vasodilatation and diuresis.

This produces a sleep that is not restful. There is no objection to taking a mild sleeping medication during the first few nights at the vacation destination. Again, taking such a medication during the flight is not recommended. Physical activity such as jogging can also positively influence adaptation.

Jet lag is not an illness, but rather an indisposition! There is no "patent remedy" to avoid it. Reasonable planning of the trip and appropriate behaviour upon arrival can shorten the duration of the symptoms!

3 Problems of adjustment to pressure changes (barotrauma)

The concept of *barotrauma* represents symptoms which are the consequence of pressure changes that occur during flight.

The symptoms usually occur soon *after leaving cruise altitude at the beginning of descent* for landing. Rarely does it occur during ascent after departure. All *gas-filled body cavities* are subject to these complaints, which usually do not result in illness. They are caused by decreasing flight altitude and increasing cabin pressure or decreasing cabin pressure and increasing flight altitude, respectively.

In rare cases these initially harmless discomforts can develop into serious symptoms of dangerous proportions that may even lead to an unplanned diversion for medical reasons. The various presentations of these conditions, including the possible ways to avoid them, are described in the following.

3.1 Ear, nose and throat

3.1.1 Maxillary sinusitis

! The maxillary sinuses are part of the stomatognathic system of the maxilla and the orbits. Therefore, the appearance of pain can be misinterpreted if one is unfamiliar with the physical/physiological relationships of this organ system, resulting in unsuccessful treatment attempts.

Lined by mucous membranes, both maxillary sinus cavities are directly connected to the middle nasal cavity through an opening. Under normal circumstances, this provides a patent canal to the outside world. *After departure* when the cabin pressure begins to decrease until the minimum cabin pressure is reached, a relative over-pressurization develops in the sinus cavities. The open windows of the middle nasal cavity may eventually prevent this, allowing the pressure to escape. The reverse relationship occurs during *descent*. Cabin pressure gradually begins to rise, as does the pressure in the sinus cavities. This process normally takes place without notice, and the passenger does not need to perform any special manoeuvres.

Disturbance of pressure equalization

Another situation arises with an otherwise harmless infection such as the common cold (rhinitis). In this case, there is a generalized swelling of the nasal mucosa, which can restrict the nasal passages. This is how *free air circulation for pressure equalization is hindered*. Corresponding symptoms almost exclusively occur *during descent*. During ascent, it is usually possible for the air to escape through these narrowed passages. The dry air during the subsequent flight increases the mucosal swelling caused by the rhinitis, leading to an increase in congestion and thereby closing off the exit passages entirely. If this pressure equalization is impeded, then the pressure inside the sinus cavities after landing is the same as at cruise altitude, approximately 1,800 m to 2,450 m. This pressure differential additionally irritates the already stressed mucosa. This results in further oedema and mucous secretion – both leading to more interference in pressure equalization. This is linked to an increasing pressure sensation all the way to severe pain, which is dull, squeezing and non-localized in nature. Because this pain can radiate from the maxillary sinuses to the area of the maxilla as well as the orbits, it can lead to a misdiagnosis of dental pain or even a non-specific process of the eye. The resulting treatments with pain medications are not directed at the cause, and are therefore often subject to failure.

Treatment is with nasal drops or sprays to reduce the mucosal swelling and allow air to freely circulate in order to equalize the pressure. The sooner treatment is begun, the faster the symptoms and complaints will resolve. The pressure sensation and pain will usually subside after one or two applications. In severe cases, reapplication in five- to ten-minute intervals may be required, depending on the intensity of the symptoms.

> A recommendation to be considered with utmost caution is the *Valsalva technique* (forcible exhalation against closed airways, mouth closed and pinching the nose shut, creating a positive pressure in the nasal/throat area in order to open the nasal sinus passage to establish equalized pressure. This may lead to a spread of bacteria to previously unaffected areas followed by a superinfection.

3.1.2   Frontal, ethmoid and sphenoid sinuses

An identical anatomical and physiological situation presents itself here, with the same therapeutic recommendations, although the pain symptoms are somewhat different in character. What they have in common is the initial pressure sensation, which worsens when bending forward or pressing.

Pain originating in the sinus frontalis is characterized by a sharp, stinging sensation; it is localized directly between the eyes ("... *like pins and needles*") and described as radiating into the head. The description is identical in the case of ethmoid sinus involvement. The sphenoid sinuses are only rarely affected, but in comparison with the previous processes the pressure here is described as dull and poorly localized intracranially, somewhat behind the orbits. Again, reduction of mucosal swelling with decongestant nasal sprays is the treatment of choice and, if begun early enough, usually brings rapid relief.

In summary, these described symptoms are annoying but still tolerable and usually do not lead to complications or permanent damage. Nonetheless, simple mucosal decongestants normally found on board every airplane can relieve the symptoms.

3.1.3   The tympanic cavity

By contrast, the symptoms, pain development and potential consequences are entirely different in the middle ear cavity. This gap within the temporal bone, which lies between the labyrinth and the tympanic membrane, contains air, is also lined by mucous membranes, and contains the fragile structures of the malleus, incus, and stapes. In order to equalize pressure, it is connected it with the external environment by the Eustachian tube which terminates in the nasopharynx. This mucosa-lined tube is composed of a bony and therefore fixed portion, and a muscular portion in the outer third that acts as a valve. It prevents, among other things, ascending infections caused by germs or viruses in the nose. Comparable to a pressure release valve, the lower portion opens in relation to pressure differentials with the outside environment. During ascent in an aircraft, travelling over mountain passes or riding in high-rise elevators, sensitive and predisposed people can experience difficulties even under normal circumstances. In the reverse direction this valve has the opposite effect in that with increasing outside pressure, pressure equalization does not occur passively, but must be actively induced. As a general rule, this is done automatically and subconsciously, but nonetheless requires active initiation.

> Activation of the throat musculature, such as by swallowing, chewing or yawning, opens the muscular component of the Eustachian tube and allows air to flow into the middle ear cavity. Of course, there is always the possibility that bacteria may ascend and result in otitis media.

In the case of infection, such as rhinitis, when the mucosal inflammation causes swelling and oedema, pressure equalization is hindered. Ascent with its corresponding pressure decrease is usually not problematic, whereas descent can be. The ventilation function of the Eustachian tube is compromised or even completely suspended. A low pressure situation develops in the middle ear cavity in relation to the external environment. The tympanic membrane's resulting inward retraction causes a pressure sensation or feeling of cotton in the ear and simultaneously reduces hearing by impairing the ability of the ear drum to vibrate, which *interferes with the proper functioning of the ossicles*. Additionally, severe *pain can rapidly develop* which is not alleviated by analgesics. After a few hours, a serous effusion can develop in the middle ear cavity resulting in a secondary middle ear infection within two days. This may result in a perforation of the tympanic membrane. However, the initial pain is already so severe that one usually seeks medical attention rather quickly.

Decongestant nasal sprays are the treatment of choice, sometimes requiring multiple and frequent applications. Nasal drops are usually more effective in infants and young children, allowing the drops to drip through the nose to the back of the throat. In this way, rapid relief can be attained. The *Valsalva manoeuvre* should be described, which was described previously: The mouth should be closed, the nose pinched shut, and pressure should be forced into the nose and throat in order to open up the sealed Eustachian tubes. Success is indicated by a crackling sensation in both ears and an immediate reduction of the feeling of numbness in the ears. If these measures are not effective, medical treatment is necessary. The first approach is to instill the appropriate nasal spray and subsequently performing the *Politzer manoeuvre*: Using a Politzer balloon, the Valsalva manoeuvre is repeated with a significantly higher pressure created by the application of the balloon. Should this fail, the only option is to perform a paracentesis as the last resort.

3.2 The lungs

It is obvious that the lungs are affected by gas expansion. In that they are an open system in constant communication with the outside atmosphere, this does not pose any problems.

> An exception exists in individuals with pulmonary emphysema. In case of larger bullae, especially those that are pleural, these can close off and, under certain circumstances, rupture. This may lead to a (tension) pneumothorax.

Under the physical conditions on board a commercial airplane, this would constitute a potentially life-threatening situation. It can occur not only in passengers but also in the crew members. The only treatment in such cases is a *rapid descent from cruise altitude* and immediate emergency landing.

> Older "frequent fliers" with corresponding medical histories are therefore encouraged to obtain the proper diagnostic work-up (see also Chapter II.5.6, Lung diseases).

3.3 Gastrointestinal tract

The effects of gastrointestinal gas expansion are of secondary importance, at least for healthy individuals. Although the absolute intraluminal volume, which is approximately 1.5 to 1.8 l, is much larger than that in the ear, nose, and throat system, the effects of intestinal distention are rare and usually do not develop into clinically significant symptoms. Due to peristalsis, the development of local accumulations of gas is unlikely. It is possible that *pressure and a feeling of fullness* can develop, as well as an upward displacement of the diaphragm in pronounced cases, but this usually does not lead to significant complaints.

In sensitive individuals, **prevention** is easy: Prior to flight, one should avoid gas-forming foods such as pulses, grain cereals, and whole wheat. The airplane meals should be chewed thoroughly and slowly, and air swallowing should be avoided. An additional, simple measure is to abstain from carbonated drinks and alcohol. Drinking too much alcohol in conjunction with mild hypoxia can have a negative effect on the intestinal peristalsis and thereby lead to gas accumulation, which can be disturbing or even painful.

4   Traveller's thrombosis

The concept of *economy class syndrome* has entered aviation medicine as a new medical condition. As it is often the case, the name is quite graphic, but does not really hit the heart of the matter. A mode of transportation, in this case the airplane, is identified as the cause of a disease even though the condition significantly precedes air travel and is only secondarily related. Because there are lawsuits pending, a brief overview is offered.

Economy class syndrome signifies a deep venous thrombosis (DVT) which may develop after relatively prolonged immobilization and may eventually lead to pulmonary embolism. The alleged cause is the seating arrangement in the airplane – hence the name! It was first described in World War I during the long stays in the trenches, and later in the Second World War among civilians who spent long periods of time in bomb shelters. Even during the 1930s there were reports regarding this phenomenon during long flights. On the whole, this condition is described repeatedly – almost always related to bus and automobile travel, but even in relation to theater events. The first controlled trial was conducted by Lufthansa German Airlines AG in 1996. The result showed that immobilization was a contributing factor, but that other aspects should be considered, such as coagulation defects and fluid imbalances. A further study at the University of Frankfurt supported these results and additionally demonstrated the influences of hypoxia, which is prevalent on board of commercial airplanes. In addition to these studies, there is a variety of other historical documentation, which cannot be proven clinically. Nonetheless, airline companies as well as the WHO are seeking additional information.

The concept of *economy class syndrome* is therefore better understood as DVT, since there is no evidence for a causal relationship with the booking class of an airline. In addition to immobility and hypoxia, other factors come into play, such as coagulation defects, varicosis with or without prior thrombosis, predisposition, medications (such as contraceptives), smoking, and alcohol consumption. The incidence of DVT is not precisely known. One can only assume that the actual figure is higher than the number of reported cases; the symptoms can appear several days after the flight, making it less likely for the traveller to connect the event with the flight.

> The present studies have resulted in a number of recommendations and countermeasures. On all Lufthansa German Airlines AG flights over 10 hours a video is shown which demonstrates in-seat isometric exercises. These exercises not only improve circulation, but also achieve a general feeling of well-being. They are also described on information cards found in the seat pockets.

For patients at risk for thrombosis there are layered recommendations. They range from wearing support stockings of the correct compression category, ingesting the right amount of fluids, avoiding long immobility, or even low-dose heparinization with low molecular weight heparin.

5 Medical conditions and flight fitness

Preface

There are only very few medical conditions that are disqualifying for air travel. With the proper planning, there are relatively few absolute medical contraindications. However, individual cases may dependent on certain equipment (such as inhalation devices, supplemental oxygen, and suction equipment) which has to be used during flight eventually disqualifying air travel.

The following describes the most common medical conditions that are relevant from the perspective of aviation physiology. The *regulations and recommendations of WHO, IATA, and AsMA* as well as the regulations of the aviation authorities will be considered in relation to admission of certain equipment on board. Specific local requirements and airport operations as well as perspectives regarding aviation security and anti-terrorism measures are not addressed. The immigration regulations of various countries with respect to the introduction of certain equipment and medications can only be broadly touched upon given that there are so many variables which can change without notice. In addition to giving consideration to the general recommendations, it is necessary to check country-specific regulations to avoid conflicts with the immigration and/or customs officials.

There is also wide range of *travel medicine information* available on the internet, often provided and regularly updated by travel medicine consultancies or pharmaceutical companies.

All medical conditions are to be evaluated individually. In the event that a number of illnesses is present, they should be evaluated in relationship to each other. Often one can determine that the underlying medical condition is negatively affected by one or more co-factors. Individually, each condition may not be of particular concern, but the combination may make air travel a challenge!

The following compilation is not only based on the frequency of inquiries by passengers or physicians, but also on incidence as reflected by the number of on-board emergencies.

> The following recommendations only apply to evaluating *medical fitness for travelling in commercial aircraft*! Secondary transport in an air ambulance follows other criteria!

5.1   Eye disorders

The eye is an organ that is minimally, if at all, affected by changes in the physical environment. Under normal circumstances there is no air- or gas-filled space in which the effects of the Boyle-Mariotte gas law can be expressed. There is, however, one significant exception that should be taken into account. Every traveller can be more or less affected by the *low humidity* and can experience itching, burning, and a foreign body sensation. Depending on individual sensitivities, *wearers of contact lenses*, especially those lenses which depend on tears to oxygenate the cornea, can be particularly impaired. In these cases it is reasonable to wear glasses during flight.

Under the conditions of mild hypoxia, there can be a slight *loss of stability of the cornea*. This is particularly important for patients who have had **laser treatments** to correct refractive errors. Depending on the extent, the cornea may be reduced by 25% of its original strength of approx. 800 μ to 650 μ. The possible reduction in visual acuity, increase in light sensitivity and worsening of astigmatism are reversible and disappear upon landing. Therefore, this bears no clinical significance for the traveller.

Poor vision, even if severe, does not play any significant aeromedical role for the traveller. It should be emphasized that an extra pair of glasses or contact lenses should be carried in the hand luggage. It is always possible that unforeseen turbulences may result in injuries from luggage falling from the overhead bins and glasses being rendered unusable.

For those with **Sjoegren's syndrome** who have sicca syndrome, it is recommended to liberally instill artificial tears; the same applies to other types of dry eyes. Facial paresis with incomplete lid closure is also important to mention. It may be necessary to instill artificial tears and tape the affected eye shut before sleeping on board in order to avoid eye dryness.

Chronic conjunctivitis may also exacerbate due to the irritation by the dry environment. Allergic conjunctivitis does not occur as the air is basically free of allergens. In the event it does occur, one should consider other causes such as food allergies and similar things.

Infectious conjunctivitis is a special situation. Normally one would not travel with this highly infectious illness. However, if it develops during a vacation, the traveller will most likely attempt to return on a regular flight. For a number of reasons, IATA regulations prohibit a traveller from flying with a communicable disease, and this type of conjunctivitis is particularly transmissible to others! This is due to the cramped confines on board, the less-than-optimal cleanliness of the washrooms, and the fact that passengers are not always very cautious about hygiene. Infectious conjunctivitis is therefore considered a reportable disease.

Retinal surgery does not set any significant limitations to flight fitness. The routine daily activities and necessities are not negatively impacted by the altered environment of the aircraft cabin. There are no other limitations following laser coagulation of the retina other than those instructions provided from an ophthalmological perspective. Similarly, there are no aeromedical concerns regarding *bioprostheses* or *silicone fillings*.

Retinal detachment, treated by a plombage sutured to the sclera to produce an indentation, also does not give rise to any particular concern. However, the application of an intraocular inert gas instillation represents a different case. Here the gas law of Boyle-Mariotte must be taken into account! The expansion of this plombage can result in compression and irreversible damage of the optic nerve!

> **Persons with intraocular gas plombage are not fit to fly!**

A bit more attention is necessary regarding **Glaucoma**. Regular treatment to reduce eye pressure is important for two reasons. The effects of time zone changes need to be taken into consideration as the chronopharmacologic conditions must be maintained within a narrow therapeutic window. As with other medical conditions, the corresponding tables obtained through travel medicine media can be used. However, the fact that travelling induces deviations from normal habits, as well as the associated stresses and numerous distractions, can make it likely to forget one's medication!

> **!** Time zone changes must be observed with glaucoma therapy!

5.2 Blood disorders

The most important consideration regarding blood disorders is the red blood cell count and haemoglobin value. What is considered to be the *normal range of Hb* varies somewhat from one airline company to another. As with many medical conditions, it depends to a certain extent on practical knowledge, from which individual cases may deviate. It is then incumbent upon the medical department of the company to make the final determination and give approval. At Lufthansa German Airlines AG, this minimum limit has been set at 9 g%.

5.2.1 Anaemia

Apart from the limits mentioned above, the cause of the anaemia must always be taken into consideration. An acute anaemia is evaluated differently than one of a chronic nature. In order to provide sufficient oxygenation to organs, particularly to the brain, an arterial saturation of 90–92% is necessary. The first symptoms appear at 85%, primarily involving the central nervous system. Vision is reduced in terms of acuity, visual fields, night vision and color discrimination. Reaction times are increased and minute motor activity is impaired. In sensitive individuals, even symptoms of *acute mountain sickness* with increasing headache and confusion can develop along with the onset of cerebral oedema. Saturations under 75% make goal-oriented activity impossible, and supplemental oxygen is the only way to reverse these symptoms, or death will occur.

Children are more sensitive to hypoxia and react more strongly than adults, resulting, for example, in severe migraine-like headaches. The reason for this difference is not known.

> **!** A minimum Hb of 9 g% has become an acceptable value!

If there are no other relevant medical conditions, such as pulmonary problems, then this value signifies adequate oxygenation and additional O_2 is not necessary. Supplemental oxygen during flight requires significant preparation and, depending on the airline, may result in substantial costs. Therefore, a careful investigation should be undertaken, including arterial blood gas analysis in case of additional complicating medical conditions.

In the event that the anaemia has been of a long-standing nature, the patient will have adapted and the acceptable limits may be more generous. This can be the case in travellers with renal insufficiency who are dependent on haemodialysis where values as low as 8–9 g% are acceptable. Similarly, this is the case for women with hypermenorrhoea with corresponding low base values. The situation is different in cases of acute anaemia such as following a gastrointestinal bleeding or trauma which do not allow for adaptation under normal circumstances and may lead to hypoxic manifestations. In such cases the patient should either wait for recovery and a normalization of the values or, if the return flight is unavoidable, receive supplemented oxygen on board of the aircraft.

> **!** Hb of 9 g% should be the guideline for determination of flight fitness!

In rare cases a blood transfusion may be recommended.

5.2.2 Thalassaemia

Thalassaemia is an exception. The two forms, thalassaemia major and minor, which occur predominantly in people of Mediterranean and Middle Eastern origin, have to be evaluated differentially.

Thalassaemia major is usually lethal in youth. Therefore, this form will only be seen in the context of an emergency repatriation flight carried out by an air ambulance organization.

Thalassaemia minor usually has an uneventful course and is generally evidenced by an elevated haemolysis and hypochromic anaemia. Treatment is generally not required as these patients have undergone adaptation. This form is also acceptable in flight crews and does not involve any limitations or special requirements.

5.2.3 Coagulation defects and anticoagulation therapy

Coagulation defects can, on the one hand, include such conditions such as traveller's thrombosis which was discussed previously, or therapeutic anticoagulation, which is described in this section. The latter is not a contraindication for flight or vacation travel! One should always evaluate the flight and the subsequent vacation or business schedule together in order to properly advise the patient.

The actual problem associated with anticoagulation treatment lies with the *underlying condition*. This must be evaluated carefully, i.e. thrombosis and embolism, coronary artery disease, or heart valve replacement.

Furthermore, passengers on anticoagulant medication should not underestimate the risk of an *injury on board*.

Consultation of patients undergoing anticoagulation should include careful advice to always fasten their seatbelts in order to avoid injury in the event of sudden turbulence!

Consultation with patients with elevated risk of bleeding should include pointing out the potential *dangers of altered behaviour during vacation*. Risks normally not taken at home are often accepted while on vacation. Tour agencies offer many sports which entail a certain risk of injury such as paragliding, tandem parachute jumping, rafting, free climbing, mountain biking, jungle excursions and the like. A further fact to consider is the increased traffic accident rate in daily life at certain vacation destinations in Africa and Asia, such as sightseeing tours and buses or the famous *Tuk-Tuks* of Thailand. Inexperienced travellers should be made aware of these situations.

Air travel and vacation are generally unhindered by anticoagulation therapy! The flight attendant should be made aware of the situation, and activity at the destination should avoid unnecessary risk!

5.3   Ear, nose and throat disorders

These usually concern simple infections which are typically ignored in daily life or are treated with home remedies or over-the-counter medications. They are therefore generally not considered significant when starting a flight even though they can lead to significant symptoms and even traumatic consequences. Fortunately this trend is noticeably decreasing as awareness of these associated problems has resulted in a widespread information campaign by the media and counseling from primary care physicians. Even so, flight reports (reports regarding incidents on board) continue to be issued regarding severe complaints on board. Although these situations do not endanger the flight or cause problems for the other passengers, the affected individual will suffer from an avoidable medical situation.

Even an obviously simple infection of the upper airways or the ear, nose and throat regions should trigger a visit to the doctor for a consultation.

5.3.1 Infections of the airways

Infections of the upper airways, ranging from harmless laryngitis to tracheitis all the way to bronchitis, do not require any special examination in terms of flight physiology. On the basis of the anatomy, there are no expected limitations beyond those that the illness entails. In this regard, a flight can be evaluated the same as any other type of travel. Either symptom severity requires cancellation of the trip, or one embarks on the flight. There is one caveat *with the elderly* if there is an associated fever over 38° C; this would raise the suspicion of other chronic lung diseases associated with a reduced gas exchange surface area such as with emphysema, chronic bronchitis, or COPD. In this case, a more detailed evaluation should be undertaken which at least involves a blood count and a determination of the peripheral oxygen saturation. In individual cases, pulmonary function tests including blood gas analysis may be necessary.

5.3.2 Rhinitis

Rhinitis, whether viral or allergic, can also be accepted. As long as there are no other anomalies, such as a significant septal deviation or otherwise hindered nasal breathing, there should not be any contraindications to flight. The timely use of a decongestant nasal spray can prevent problems caused by pressure disequilibrium.

5.3.3 Sinusitis

Sinusitis or pansinusitis must be evaluated carefully. In an uncomplicated situation, the pressure differences can usually be managed without any problems as long as a nasal spray is used. During descent, it should be instilled at 10- to 15-minute intervals until landing (see also Chapter II.3, Problems of adjustment to pressure changes).

In the event that rhinitis is also present – which is often the case! – it is important to evaluate the situation more carefully.

Chronic (pan)sinusitis is not amenable to decongestant therapy. If significant symptoms exist and there is a desire or need to fly frequently, then a surgical procedure or intervention may be considered.

5.3.4 Otitis media

Care and caution are recommended when acute or chronic otitis media is present, particularly when dealing with infants and young children! The narrow tympanic cavity is unable to equalize pressure at ground level and the gradual resorption of air is virtually impossible. In addition to a reduction in hearing, significant pain can develop at various intensities. Even liberal applications of decongestant cannot relieve the swelling of the inflamed and oedematous mucosa. The Eustachian tubes thus become dysfunctional and can no longer equalize the subnormal pressure. These painful symptoms would significantly worsen when exposed to further pressure differentials.

Acute otitis media is therefore disqualifying for flight until complete recovery! It is also one of the rare medical conditions which is refundable (with medical documentation) under travel cancellation insurance. This requires a functional evaluation of the Eustachian tubes, such as by tympanometry, performed by an ENT physician!

! Acute otitis media is a contraindication for air travel!

5.4 Heart and circulatory disorders

As with many other medical conditions of entire organ systems, cardiovascular diseases require the evaluation of certain parameters in every case. Likewise, it is necessary to identify comorbidities. Especially limitations in daily life activities need to be considered.

The following diagnostic steps may be undertaken considering flight fitness:

1. **Laboratory**: Small bloodcount, electrolytes
2. **ECG**: Resting ECG, stress testing for CAD
3. **Lungs**: Vital capacity, FEV_1, peripheral oximetry

In individual cases, (stress) echocardiography, Holter monitoring or 24-hour blood pressure measurements may be useful.

5.4.1 Arterial hypertension

According to the WHO definitions, there are four stages of blood pressure which range from borderline to severe hypertension:

- Borderline hypertension
  90 to 94 mmHg (diastolic)
- Mild hypertension
  95 to 109 mmHg (diastolic)
- Intermediate hypertension
  110 to 114 mmHg (diastolic)
- Severe hypertension
  over 115 mmHg (diastolic)

Conditions caused by pressure changes, such as hypoxia, require relatively rapid compensatory mechanisms of the body which should be considered not only when evaluating hypertension, but also with regard to other cardiovascular conditions such as cardiac insufficiency or CAD.

The healthy person increases the depth and rate of breathing, and a slight increase in heart rate can be observed. By increasing ventilation and raising cardiac output, hypoxia is thus minimized and saturation is maintained at 94–96%. Simultaneously, through adrenergic mechanisms, blood vessels in the pulmonary circulation system contract, increasing pressure by 5–10 mmHg. These physiological reactions are tolerable for healthy individuals, but not always for people with acute or chronic medical problems.

Neither borderline nor hypertension require any special evaluation if well controlled with medications and free of impairing side effects. There should be no secondary organ system problems that need to be taken into consideration. Sudden hypertensive crises are not to be expected, and even with mildly elevated blood pressure, there is no significant problem associated with time zone changes and subsequent irregular medication intake.

Intermediate hypertension can result in physiological reactions that may increase the load on the circulatory system and lead to elevated blood pressure. Even when this is expected, the effect may not necessarily be so serious as to lead to a hypertensive crisis. As long as the medications are taken regularly and the time zone changes are taken into consideration so that there is no drop below therapeutic levels, no further precautions should be necessary. Only the general guidelines for on-board care apply.

Severe hypertension requires particular attention regarding the (not uncommon) condition of arterial hypertension. Usually there are also associated medical conditions which can worsen the overall medical situation.

> Prior to flight, careful attention must be given to blood pressure management and a change in medications made if required!

5.4.2 Pulmonary hypertension

Pulmonary hypertension per se is no contraindication for flying; also mild hypoxia in cruising altitude will – irrespective of the underlying cause of pulmonary hypertension – further increase pulmonary artery pressure. The ultimate criteria for "fitness to fly" are the ability of the right section of the heart to compensate for the increasing pressure. I.e. it still has to shift blood through the lungs without right heart congestion or even failure.

Patients with severe pulmonary hypertension and chronic anticoagulation who take any specific drugs (such as sildenafil or iloprost) to decrease their pulmonary pressure require close attention by an experienced pulmonologist and assessment by an aviation medicine specialist.

> Travelling by air may well lead to decompensation in such patients and this may therefore require close attention.

5.4.3 Congestive heart failure

Fully compensated and well-controlled cardiac insufficiency is not a contraindication for air travel. This results in full adaptation without the risk of decompensation.

With regard to flight duration, a sufficient fluid balance is mandatory. Although the dry cabin air should be taken into consideration, the likelihood of peripheral edema is still increased, given the low ambient pressure. By this, the risk of acute cardiac failure due to volume overload is increased considerably. For this reason, the use of non-alcoholic beverages like water or juices is preferred.

> Careful control of fluid balance is suggested.

Prophylaxis of oedema and improvement of well-being can be achieved by performing regular isometric exercises and muscle stretching, both of which can be accomplished while seated without releasing the seat belt. Tutorials are found in the flight information packet and in the seat-back instructions.

Medications can be managed within the accustomed regimen and adapted to the new time zone with minimal difficulty.

5.4.4 Coronary artery disease

Evaluation of coronary artery disease is one of the most common issues in daily medical practice. There are two reasons which necessitate careful judgment. On the one hand, there are the interests of the traveller. Depending on the stage of disease and the physical requirements while on board the aircraft, a *determination of risk* must be made. Additionally, there are the aspects of flight safety and the avoidance of undue inconvenience to the other passengers which can result from unscheduled landings due to medical problems.

In order to characterize the functional limitations induced by coronary artery disease the international established CCS-score (Canadian Cardiovascular Society) is easy to apply and with its four categories comparable all over the world. Regardless of the severity of the functional limitations or the CCS-class, some recommendations remain unchanged: the CCS-score allows us to illustrate criteria for "fitness to fly" with underlying coronary artery disease:

- **CCS stage 0/I**: no clinical signs or symptoms during daily life and thereby no restriction during daily activities. No symptoms at rest and no chronic drug therapy. Thus, there is here unrestricted "fitness to fly" and no precautionary measures are applicable.
- **CCS stage II**: during strain or stress symptoms like chest pain, nitro-positive. Patient's awareness with regard to onset of signs and symptoms of coronary artery disease needs to be raised. Prompt drug therapy and supplemental oxygenation is indicated.
- **CCS stage III**: light activity already induces chest pain or equivalent signs or symptoms of coronary artery disease. Cabin altitude of 1,800 to 2,450 m may already lead during rest to insufficient oxygenation of the myocardium and consequently to chest pain and cell damage.
- **CCS stage IV**: this is characterized by the existence of angina at rest, i.e. the so-called unstable angina.

Here, flight approval can only be obtained under special circumstances. In each case, *continuous supplemental oxygen* is necessary in order to achieve sufficient oxygen saturation at rest.

Often, angina is the first manifestation of underlying coronary artery disease which develops when one is aboard. In such cases the flight back home may be feasible given specific circumstances; here, an accompanying physician and supplemental oxygen supply is required. Eventual angina may be relieved by drug therapy.

Under normal circumstances, even sitting at rest with supplemental oxygen and **accompanied by a physician,** this may not be possible. Often the only option is supine transport on a **stretcher** (installed in a commercial aircraft), as long as there are no other associated medical conditions and pulmonary function and haemoglobin are generally normal. In this manner, circulatory stress is minimized and intravenuos infusion and circulatory support is possible.

For particularly difficult cases, the **PTC**, or **patient transport compartment** may be utilized. This involves a special cabin which can be installed into a variety of widebody aircraft, making it possible to deliver intensive medical care including controlled artificial breathing.

Recommendations for coronary heart disease

CCS Class 0/I: *No limitations*
CCS Class II: *Consultation prior to travel*
CCS Class III: *Special consideration necessary*
CCS Class IV: *Transport only as an exceptional case with appropriate equipment*

5.4.5   Cardiac dysrhythmia

Apart from its clinical significance, cardiac dysrhythmia must be evaluated for flight fitness in each case with regard to mild *hypoxia* even if it is fully compensated. As with other medical conditions, and not only in the cardio-vascular realm, optimal treatment and stability are necessary, but there should also be no complicating comorbidities.

As a general rule, with good control, there are no specific requirements!

5.4.6   Pacemakers

No specific precautions are necessary for individuals with pacemakers or automatic defibrillators.

Today's implanted devices are protected against electromagnetic interference and neither the metal detectors at airport security checkpoints nor the electronic aircraft systems disturb them. The electromagnetic fields are so minimal that pacemakers are not adversely affected. This also applies to the seemingly older metal detector gates at some airports. The avionic systems themselves are so well protected from external influences that they neither impact pacemakers nor are negatively affected by them.

5.4.7   Valvular heart disease/Congenital heart disease

Congenital heart disease, with its variable haemodynamic effects and re-lated oxygenation impairments, must be carefully assessed individually. In the case of the adult, one can assume either that the congenital defect is not severe, or that he or she has undergone adaptation and compensation over the years. Valvular heart disease is frequently found in adults, and often already surgically corrected or without clinical relevance. Thus, no require-ments with regard to fitness to fly apply with one exception: dyspnea or signs and symptoms of cardiac decompensation with minimal exertion at sea level.

5.4.8 Inflammatory heart diseases/Endocarditis

Inflammatory diseases of the myocardium, epicardium, or valves lead to variable limitations of cardiac performance and corresponding secondary organ damage from hypoxia due to reduced perfusion. This leads to the risk of clinically significant and *malignant cardiac dysrhythmias* and *decompensation*.

> Absolutely no flight is possible during the acute phase of inflammatory heart disease. Rest and avoidance of any type of stress to the heart is indicated.

After recovery, as a general rule, there are no further limitations as long as function has been restored with no heart blocks, dysrhythmias, or reduction in cardiac output. In these cases, evaluation should be based on the aforementioned criteria.

5.5 Infectious diseases

National regulations

As long as travel between countries and continents has existed, the various conveyances have also paved the way for worldwide distribution of diseases. In the past, entire continents were overrun by completely and unknown new epidemics. One only needs to recall measles on the American continent or the spread of the plague in Europe. In both these cases ships were the vehicle and the carriers were humans or animals. Protective measures at the time included the establishment of quarantine. Ships arriving from countries with serious epidemics or with cases of acute illness on board were required to wait at sea for 40 days without any contact. If no further cases appeared on board, the ship was allowed to enter the port.

Air travel today, with approximately two billion (2,000,000,000) passengers annually worldwide, has, of course, significantly reduced transmission time for epidemics. One can be thankful that epidemics can be controlled by local measures and outbreaks contained. Nonetheless, the most recent events remind us of the problem. Periodically there are massive outbreaks of local epidemics in Africa, such as Ebola or Lassa fever. Albeit quite unlikely, it is entirely possible that an asymptomatic yet ill traveller may spread a disease worldwide. The outbreak of the plague in India in 1994 required significant time- and energy-intensive resources to prevent importation. The situation was even more critical after the outbreak of SARS in 2002, and with the emergence of avian influenza (H5N1) in 2003. A further example, which has not received the same level of attention, is the West Nile virus, brought to the previously unaffected North American continent by visitors from the Near East in 1999. In the course of a few years it spread to the west coast of the US. The latest event was the swine flu, or new flu, spreading across the globe from Mexico in April 2009 within just a few months.

It should be emphasized that the airplane is merely the transport vehicle – the carriers are always people or animals. This is also the case with the extremely rare, so-called *airport malaria*. It occurs when malaria-infested Anopheles mosquitoes are transported in the cargo hold or cabin and cause malaria infections at destinations where the disease normally does not exist.

> *Since there is variability among countries regarding prophylaxis, disinsection and disinfection measures should be undertaken before and during flight prior to landing. Examination of passengers is not routinely performed. Infectious tuberculosis is an exception, in accordance with WHO recommendations. In some countries follow-up examinations of other passengers must be performed – see for special national regulations!*

General recommendations

Member airlines of IATA have a general duty of care toward their passengers. These requirements are defined by the *Warsaw Convention* of 1929, which is still valid today and encompasses the minimization of certain specified health impairments.

The risk of infection on board an aircraft is much lower than on other comparable means of transportation, such as rail or coach, or on mass transit vehicles such as commuter trains or buses. The otherwise unpleasant effects of the air conditioning system, i.e. very dry air and a high air exchange rate, are actually beneficial! They significantly reduce the infectiousness of bacteria and viruses which can be transmitted by droplet spread. The rest is eliminated by the HEPA filters. It is not possible to prevent direct person-to-person infection which occurs between passengers in neighbouring seats. A distance of about two rows in front of and behind the infected person, as well as two seats to either side, can be assumed to be a realistic distance for droplet spread to occur. Additionally, movement of the ill passenger within the aircraft, such as through the aisle to the washroom and waiting in line with other passengers, can promote further spread.

In the event that a pertinent case becomes known, the appropriate measures must be taken. These are based in part on the recommendations of the WHO but must also follow the regulations of the countries involved. All of the at-risk passengers and crew must be informed, whereas the ground crew is not necessarily included. Passengers within the aforementioned range of the ill person are advised to see a doctor, and, if necessary, may be ordered to do so. The same applies to the cabin crew who worked within range. The airline must notify the local public health authorities by providing the passenger and crew manifests. In addition, the medical departments of the airline may issue further recommendations.

5.5.1 Measles, chickenpox, and pertussis

> Individuals with these and other common childhood infectious diseases are restricted from travelling until the infectious period has ended!

In general, patients are not significantly impaired. The associated fever additionally increases the hypoxia-induced, slightly elevated heart rate. The same is true for the respiratory rate. Combined with an elevated body temperature, this may lead to significant dehydration. These children or patients respectively therefore need special attention to increase their fluid intake.

There exists an increased risk of infection transmission because flights generally involve several hours on board combined with the close quarters and direct contact with other passengers.

5.5.2 Tuberculosis

Tuberculosis, while occurring worldwide, particularly in countries with reduced living and sanitary standards, has largely receded into the background in European countries. Through intensive air travel, however, it is becoming more evident even there. For the purposes of travel medicine, the discussion is limited to pulmonary tuberculosis.

> An ill person with open and therefore infectious tuberculosis must not be transported!

This recognition absolutely presents a problem. Diagnosis of the illness results in air travel restriction. Unknown are those who either disregard their medical consultation or those who do not yet recognize their illness. Closed tuberculosis does not affect other passengers or crew. Air or gas inclusions in encapsulated lesions may, however, expand according to the gas law of *Boyle-Mariotte* and rupture. If this occurs close to the pleura, it can lead to a *pneumothorax* and may rapidly become life-threatening on board. Perforation into the bronchia and trachea may result in exposure of other passengers due to droplet spread.

5.5.3 HIV infection

Due to the threat of other epidemics, HIV, like tuberculosis, has dropped out of the focus of public interest.

> For air travel, HIV does not impose any limitations, as there is no increased risk for the other passengers on board.

Attention should be given to the entry requirements of various countries which either may require health certificates or even a test on arrival as a condition of entry, particularly for extended stays. It is therefore very important to have the appropriate tests performed in advance. In that the requirements can change quickly, it is recommended that up-to-date information is obtained through the various travel medicine media.

> HIV infection requires review of the current entry requirements!

5.5.4 Hepatitis

Chronic and clinically compensated Hepatitis B and C as well as D and E do not pose any risk for affected passengers or bystanders such as fellow passengers or crew. In contrast, acute Hepatitis A and E may be transmitted – regardless of clinical signs and symptoms – by oral or fecal routes. Therefore a theoretical risk exists for fellow passengers or crews sharing wash rooms or toilets on board of the aircraft. Thus appropriate modes of disinfection not only for hands but also for all surfaces in question have to be in place.

5.5.5 MRSA

Increasingly, questions arise regarding flight acceptability while infected with or following MRSA infection. Since *Methicillin-resistant staph. aureus infections* are occurring in hospitals more and more frequently, air ambulances are more and more often asked by physicians to transport MRSA patients.

Therefore the problem occurs after the infection has subsided. Transmission occurs by droplets and fomites. The use of protective equipment, such as a mask, is generally sensible but creates undue fear among the other passengers that usually can not be alleviated by any amount of explanation. The risk of fomite transmission is certainly heightened due to the less than optimal sanitary conditions on board (small washrooms, heavy use by passengers with varying hygienic standards).

> **!** Air travel is only possible after complete resolution of MRSA!

5.5.6 Ebola and Lassa fever

These African diseases, with their high infectivity and lethality, are obviously not allowed to travel on commercial airplanes in any situation. It is quite unusual that a flight is requested after the illness has manifested. In contrast is the situation where *the illness is discovered after an infected passenger has flown*. As with tuberculosis, there is a requirement to provide passenger information as well as to perform examinations. Additionally, the *aircraft* must be *disinfected*, a costly and time-consuming endeavor.

5.6 Lung diseases

Introduction

All pulmonary diseases must be evaluated according to certain basic principles. The first one is *Dalton's law*. It determines arterial oxygen saturation in relation to the ambient pressure and thus for the partial O_2 pressure. An elevation of 5,500 m reduces the total pressure by half to 380 mmHg with a corresponding partial oxygen pressure of 92 mmHg. In reference to the average cabin pressure of 550 mmHg, this corresponds to an O_2 partial pressure of 102 mmHg. This reduces the base value of oxygenation to 61%. Furthermore, many people with pulmonary diseases have a thickened membrane in the area between alveoli and capillaries – a situation which is often underappreciated and further compromises oxygenation. Equally important is the total ventilatory surface area, as well as other factors such as pH, CO_2 pressure in the blood, body temperature, and adrenaline levels due to stressful situations. This results in some basic diagnostic steps which are necessary in each individual case. All pulmonary cases should be evaluated in advance with these issues in mind. Certain individual cases may require further steps.

Fundamentals of lung disease diagnosis

- Peripheral O_2 saturation, pulse oxymetry
- Walking distance, 6 minute walking test
- requirement of oxygen at home

Andvanced diagnostics, only if clinically indicated

- Lung funktion test
- Blood gas analysis
- Hb-Level
- Chest x-ray or CT

5.6.1 Bronchial asthma

Bronchial asthma belongs to the class of pulmonary diseases that require the greatest amount of consultation. Among actual medical events on board, asthma exacerbations are ranking on the eight place of the statistic, behind the commonly encountered cardiovascular problems and injuries! A *qualified prior consultation* significantly reduces complications during travel!

> **!** In general there are no objections, given proper precautions!

The minimum necessities for lung function should of course be provided. Additional aspect to keep in mind include *the avoidance of stressful situations* and the avoidance of physical overexertion. Stress reduction should include, for example, arriving at the airport with enough time to go through security. The luggage should consist of several bags rather than one very large suitcase and the help of porters should be enlisted.

Carry-on luggage should contain *adequate amounts of the required medication* to last through the first week. Additionally, one must be prepared for a sudden bronchospasm by carrying a rapid-onset broncholytic.

> *In the airplane, one should be aware of certain environmental factors.*

Exposure to very dry air on longer flights may irritate the air passages and initiate an acute attack. Improvement by *humidifying the air* can be achieved by breathing through the nose, which must of course be unobstructed, and by moistening the nasal mucosa with sprays or gels that contain physiological saline. Not to be underestimated are *stress* triggers in the airplane such as cramped seats or an unpleasant neighbour.

Some toxic chemicals used to exist in the cabin air, such as tobacco smoke, which thankfully is no longer a factor since all flights are now non-smoking, and ozone, contained in the outside air, is kept out of the cabin by catalytic converters.

Attack-inducing allergens are also not found in cabin air thanks to the well-designed filtration technology and high air exchange rates with a maximum proportion of recycled air of 45%. Not entirely controllable, some components of catering or particularly strong perfumes of neighbouring passengers may be *allergenic*.

5.6.2 Bronchitis

Acute bronchitis does not necessarily require cancellation of the flight if it is very difficult or not possible to change the ticket. The limitation of lung function is not severe in these cases, and the unfavorable physical/physiological factors have little clinical significance. One must be mindful of the dry air and there should be adequate moisturizing of the mucous membranes.

> With chronic bronchitis, it is assumed that the patient is accustomed to the symptoms and that the dry air does not have a significant irritating effect.

5.6.3 COPD – Chronic obstructive pulmonary disease

Because the age of passengers is increasing, especially those who are tourists or use charter flights, COPD is occurring more frequently. Many patients in this group aim to flee the European winter and spend the cold season on the Balearic or Canary Islands or even in the Caribbean.

> *While a short flight to the Mediterranean only rarely requires much in the way of precautionary measures,* **long-haul flights** *can present quite a different challenge!*
>
> *In the majority of cases, supplemental oxygen is required at least intermittently during the day and/or continuously during sleep!*

Less commonly, there are those who will require uninterrupted portable supplemental O_2. These patients may be adapted to a life at sea level with minimal oxygenation but decompensate when in the airplane. Here they will *require constant supplemental* O_2, often with high flow rates. If a continuous supply of supplemental oxygen is required, the Wenoll System as well as a number of portable oxygen concentrators chosen from various companies may fulfill the needs. More than ten such systems have been cleared by various authorities for the use during flight. Nevertheless, details shall be negotiated with the particular airline.

Of note is the power source for such devices. Some airlines claim that life-sustaining equipment has to be usable independent of power sources of the aircraft since these cannot be guaranteed for example in case of turbine failure. By regulation, their batteries must be sufficient in number and charge to run the system for 150% of the estimated flight time, e.g. for a ten hour flight, 15 hours of energy need to be offered. Moreover, one has to be aware that energy consumption of oxygen concentrators dramatically increases with increasing oxygen/flow demands!

5.6.4 Emphysema

The main concern regarding pulmonary emphysema is the reduced surface area for gas exchange due to overinflation. Additionally, increased membrane thickness resulting in a reduction of diffusion capacity must be considered.

> It is recommended that the lower limit for peripheral oxygen saturation should be maintained at 90% to 92% under normal circumstances.

> Lower values require at least intermittent supplemental oxygen and should be managed by way of pulse oximetry.

5.6.5 Pneumonia

Suffering from acute pneumonia an individual is by definition unfit to fly. Under specific circumstances, a transport utilizing the PTC may be feasible in the acute setting.

Even after a case of pneumonia and relief of all symptoms, patients should still rest for a couple of days – depending on age, comorbidities and functional limitations – prior to boarding a flight. Together with functional capacity of an individual, the duration of the desired flight has to be considered: a one-hour continental flight should not pose any problems early after a case of pneumonia, in contrast to a twelve hour long-haul, intercontinental flight.

> *Should a flight be necessary, e.g. illness in a foreign country resulting in a protracted treatment, then a repatriation flight can be undertaken using a stretcher or PTC. In this way, necessary intensive therapeutic measures such as intravenous infusion, antibiotic medications, circulatory support, suctioning and control of secretions, fluids and electrolyte balance, or O_2 ventilation, etc., can be provided.*

5.6.6 Pneumothorax

> An acute pneumothorax is an absolute contraindication to flight, without exception!

Even in military circumstances with significantly more generous criteria, this necessitates ground transportation. Transport by helicopter may be considered whereby flight levels above 300 m would not be exceeded. The now inflated pleural space may lead to compression against the mediastinum, resulting in cardiovascular as well as pulmonary compromise. Through the reduction of the ambient pressure, the situation can be significantly worsened by gas expansion according to the *Boyle-Mariotte gas law*. This is a set-up for a lethal outcome from total cardiovascular collapse!

When is flight possible after a pneumothorax?

Since there are no official guidelines, only recommendations based on individual case assessment can be offered as long as the intent of the *Warsaw Convention* is observed. In general, four to six weeks of convalescence is usually adequate to assume stable conditions and flight is no longer contraindicated. Of course, the patient's history is very important. A first-time episode with an obvious cause is more likely to be assessed favourably with respect to flying. Multiple relapses or a diagnosis of pleural bullae carrying a risk of rupture which may lead to further episodes necessitate a more stringent position. These passengers require consultation regarding surgical intervention or must forgo flight for the rest of their lives.

5.7   Gastrointestinal disorders

Gastrointestinal diseases generally do not represent a primary restriction for flying. However, accompanying symptoms, such as bleeding ulcers with significant secondary anaemia, may result in disqualification.

> Absolute contraindications include ileus as well as sub-ileal symptoms and uncontrollable diarrhea!

Other chronic illnesses, such as regional ileitis or Crohn's disease, normally are not limiting. However, the patient should be aware of travel stressors, like adapting to time zone changes and an unfamiliar diet and the fact that these factors may precipitate acute episodes even in those patients who are otherwise well controlled and in full remission of their illness.

5.8 Neurological disorders

5.8.1 General guidelines

Neurological disorders only rarely require aeromedical evaluation, as they generally are not affected by flight. The primary criteria here have to do with the comfort of the other passengers and the *undisturbed operation of the flight*. From this perspective, the duties of the cabin crew should be reviewed.

> **The cabin crew**
>
> Their primary responsibility is for safety on board. This begins with the preparation and supervision of the cabin and includes control of the passengers regarding regulations and first aid in medical emergencies, and ends with emergency landing and evacuation. Secondarily they provide cabin service, which is what the passengers observe and therefore may create a false impression of the cabin crew's task. It is definitely not their duty to provide care to a passenger as a personal attendant when it is obvious that the passenger is not in a position to care for him- or herself.

Neurological and psychiatric illnesses are often recognized by the fact that they require assistance for simple functions. This can be the case for paralysis when an immobilized patient is not able to fasten the seat belt or use the toilet. There may be psychological disturbances that make communication impossible, or psychiatric illnesses with delusions that result in unusual, if not dangerous, behaviour that is not controllable. For these reasons, illnesses in these two categories *always require a competent attendant* who serves as a connection to the more or less foreign outside world. This attendant must not only have the proper training to manage the psychological condition, but also be able to manage the necessary activities of daily living.

Neurological illnesses often require a (medical) escort!

A further requirement which the afflicted as well as the support groups often do not appreciate is that every air passenger must be able to follow through with instructions regarding safety requirements. This may be impossible for the paraplegic and lead to being required – often not understandable for the person in question – to reserve a stretcher.

Parents with handicapped children often want to utilize the car seat that the hospital has provided. Again, due to special technical considerations, these are usually not allowed because, although they can be fastened in by the seat belt they may not be able to be unbuckled properly. In contrast to the push-button releases used in automobile seat belts, those used in aircraft are flap locks and there may not be enough space to release them when the arm rests are locked in the downward position.

5.8.2 Neurological conditions with physical limitations

Quite often, neurological conditions are combined with physical limitations. The spectrum ranges from motor restrictions to incontinence, to speech and mental disorders. The challenge here is to find a *solution in accordance with the physical symptom*. On the one hand, there is a desire to accommodate the afflicted person and make them as comfortable as possible. On the other hand, there are limitations when the measures are so cumbersome that they are not technically feasible due to space and equipment requirements. The evaluation must take into consideration that commercial airlines are a means of conveyance, not air ambulances. Limits are also set with regard to the comfort of other passengers, a factor often forgotten by the evaluating physicians. What is medically possible is not always feasible.

Regarding disabled passengers, please also see Chapter II.9.

5.9 Psychiatric disorders

Preface

Psychiatric disorders have a special role in medical evaluation. While the Warsaw Convention assessed not only the rights but also the general responsibilities of passengers, the IATA criteria mainly relate to recommendations concerning flight fitness and can therefore be variably interpreted and applied by the airlines. The situation is further complicated by the fact that within the Anglo-American realm, even mild-depression can fall under these definitions. Historically linked to the beginnings of commercial aviation, this view is not supported in today's medical practice, yet the definition remains unchanged. For this reason, airline companies have found a variety of solutions.

The following is the *interpretation of Lufthansa German Airlines AG*, which may differ from that of other airline companies.

5.9.1 Depression

Aviation medicine does not differentiate between endogenous and exogenous depression, and there are no aeromedical aspects to be taken into consideration. Depending on the situation and orientation capabilities of the patient, flight may certainly be undertaken alone. If necessary, an *attendant service* is available to manage check-in, customs and passport formalities, and also bring the patient to the airplane, explain the special circumstances to the flight attendants and provide further instructions. At the destination the opposite procedure takes place ending with handover to those picking up the passenger.

As previously noted, a trip can be a thoroughly *stressful situation*. Many factors can lead to a deteriorating mood. The treating physician should first confirm that the medication is *dosed properly*. Similarly, it is especially important to confirm that the antidepressant medications have been taken regularly.

5.9.2   Psychosis

> **!** Acute psychosis is an absolute contraindication for commercial flights!

Oftentimes, the following situation occurs: A patient with a psychosis and well controlled on medication, is symptom-free, and clinically doing well. He does not undergo consultation prior to travelling because he is feeling well. During his vacation he neglects to take his psychiatric medication regularly, partly because of the time zone shift. He develops an acute *exacerbation*, perhaps even violent behavior, is arrested, and ends up as a patient in a psychiatric clinic – a bad situation in a foreign country with language barriers, medication or other problems. After improvement, he wishes to fly back home; unfortunately, this is contrary to regulations!

Return flight after acute psychosis

The *return flight* is still possible but only under certain *binding conditions* which cannot be deviated from! First of all, adequate remission with stable conditions must be reached. The flight can then take place *accompanied by a physician*, usually a specialist in psychiatry or neurology. The attending physician must be in the position to manage the patient medically during the flight. Possibly, a second assistant with psychiatric experience may be required! In any case, safety and an undisturbed flight is the highest priority. For this reason, it is sometimes necessary for a longer period of stability to have passed before flight approval can be given.

> ✈ *Travellers with psychosis must be accompanied by a physician in any case, and an additional assistant may be necessary!*

5.10   Kidney disorders

Chronic kidney diseases are usually associated with hypertension and anaemia. The evaluation therefore generally takes these two conditions into consideration.

Dialysis patients are in general adapted to their anaemia, and the aforementioned Hb of 9 g% can be a used as a guide. However, should it fall below 7.5%, a transfusion is indicated prior to travel.

Due to the continuous technical improvement of dialysis, especially the introduction of CAPD (*continuous ambulatory peritoneal dialysis*) and the development of dialysis centres at vacation destinations, these patients have become increasingly mobile and can travel almost worldwide. With CAPD, the dialysis fluid remains in the intraperitoneal cavity for four to six hours before it is removed. This allows patients to be nearly self-sufficient with unlimited mobility. There is no problem if on occasion the fluid is not replaced for eight or ten hours, which may be the case for long-haul flights. *Removal of dialysis fluid during flight* is not possible due to the physical constraints and less than optimal hygienic conditions in the washrooms. It is recommended to interrupt the trip for one or two days, which is also favourable for the circadian rhythm. Many tour operators already offer such "stop-over programmes" for flights to the Far East and Australia. The only question then is how to transport the rather large amount of required dialysis fluid if it is not available at the destination. Many airlines have special regulations regarding transport of certain types of luggage. It is therefore possible that the transport may be without charge or for a reduced fee for the excess luggage as it is a medical necessity. However, one should inquire about this with each individual airline.

> Like all patients with chronic medical conditions, dialysis patients should carry with them their medical records (preferably in English). In the case of an emergency in a foreign country, this will facilitate appropriate treatment.

5.11 Metabolic disorders

Preface

Many metabolic disorders require continuous medication in regular intervals. Often there are corresponding dietary restrictions. The main focus is on the time zone change with the associated therapeutic adjustment. In addition, it is necessary to request the appropriate special diet on the airplane. An understanding of the choices and the processes ensures that the required meals are provided even on very long flights. Using international notation codes, this system functions smoothly among IATA member airlines.

Lufthansa German Airlines AG provides about 25 so-called *Special Meals*. This is entirely comparable to what is provided at nutrition clinics for patients with metabolic disorders. *Catering* generally requires a minimum 24-hour notification in advance of the flight. Table 8 describes these *Special Meals* that are either required or recommended with regards to metabolic physiology.

Tab. 8   Special Meals of Lufthansa German Airlines AG

Internat. Code	Type of meal	Description
BLML	Bland Soft Meal	Light meal for stomach, bowels, liver and gall bladder
DBML	Diabetic Meal (two versions)	Special meal for diabetes; no sugar, low fat, no breaded food, non alcoholic
GFML	Gluten-free Meal	Meal for those allergic to gluten; no wheat, rye, barley, oat, flour products /souces
HFML	High Fibre Meal	Meal with nutritious value, fresh base products
LCML	Low Calory Meal	Meal with reduced calories, plenty of roughage, low in fat and carbohydrates
LFML	Low Cholesterol Meal	Special meal for metabolic disease; less than 100 mg cholesterol per meal; no animal fats, no egg yolk
LPML	Low Protein Meal	Low protein and low sodium meal for sickness of liver
LSML	Low Sodium Meal	Alt-free meal for heart, circulation, kidneys; low fat, non-flatulent, low on liquid, non-alcoholic
NLML	No Lactose/ No Lacto-Meal	Meal for those allergic to milk or suffering from lactose intolerance
PRML	Low Purin Meal	Meal with low uiric acid content (no offal)

These 15 diet types are mostly ordered for the corresponding disorder or to accommodate certain nutritional choices. In addition, there are *10 Special Meals* which can accommodate specific eating habits or meet religious food requirements. Thus, not only vegetarians but also vegans can be provided their meals of choice without having to pick through their food. A Muslim may receive appropriately prepared meals just as a rabbi may be served a kosher meal with the assurance that the requirements were observed.

5.11.1   Diabetes mellitus

The most significant of the metabolic disorders is diabetes. The occurence of type 1 and 2 in about 4% of the general population makes this an increasingly common encountered disease on board. For these travellers, the trip begins much earlier than with the start of the flight.

Already a few weeks in advance, one should pay attention to one's metabolic condition. Documentation of daily blood glucose profiles should be discussed with the treating physician. In this manner, abnormal values can be ascertained and improvements made in self-medication. In order to avoid hypoglycaemic episodes *one should not attempt extremely tight control*.

Particular attention should be paid to potential comorbidities. These should be accurately determined, medications reviewed and, if necessary, changed or readjusted. It is also possible that patients are counselled against taking the trip even though each individual medical condition may be considered safe for flight, as the summation of the problems may potentiate the risk of a medical incident.

Security checks, syringe, pen or injector

Due to today's heightened security measures the fact that insulin is injected by syringes, pens, or injectors increases the likelihood of problems at airports. General guidelines cannot be provided since these requirements are country-specific and are implemented locally. The airlines do not have any influence in this area. The security personnel is not necessarily knowledgeable on the topic or flexible, and the situation may be exacerbated by the inability to communicate in the local language. Syringes may be considered weapons and be confiscated. What is even worse is if the syringes are interpreted by the authorities as instruments of illegal drug use. As with other medical conditions, it is worth repeating that the corresponding medical certificate regarding the necessity of the medical treatment – preferably in English – should be carried by the passenger. In the interest of the traveller, this recommendation should be considered to be a requirement. It would be negligent to go without it!

Patients with insulin pumps will find it somewhat easier. The material to fill the ports can be carried in the checked luggage and will not cause security problems. Of course, the metal detectors at the security checkpoints will trigger an alarm. The necessary medical certificate with illustrations and pictures can easily clarify the situation. In this regard, American medicine is somewhat more advanced not only with respect to the simplification of air travel but also as far as security check points are concerned. Many people with implanted devices, such as insulin pumps and pacemakers or prosthetic knee or hip joints, carry a special card with personal data, photographs, and radiographs of the corresponding region. This clarifies the situation for the security personnel and eliminates the problem.

Security issues with personal medical supplies can lead to significant delays if it is necessary to repack some of the medical supplies from the hand bags to the checked luggage so that syringes, etc. can be taken along but are inaccessible on board. In order to not miss the flight, it is best to plan on taking more time at the point of departure and also during transfers or layovers. However, a portion should always remain in the carry-on luggage as there is always the possibility that the checked luggage is misplaced or not transferred due to insufficient time and therefore does not arrive at the destination until several days later, if at all.

Insulin adjustment

During the flight, attention should be paid to begin adjusting the insulin regimen to the time zone of the destination, *taking meal service into account.*

> *An important rule to follow in the airplane is that insulin should not be injected before the meal has been served!*

Unanticipated events, such as turbulence, can interrupt meal service or cancel it altogether. If the insulin has already been injected and there is no snack available either, then a hypoglycaemic episode is guaranteed to follow. One should always have an emergency ration, perhaps in the form of glucose, *readily available in the hand luggage.*

In general, westward flights require an additional insulin injection due to the lengthening of the day. The reverse is true for eastward flights, where the dose should be reduced. There are insulin tables available on the internet from various travel medicine information sites. Here one can enter the flight data, times and the type and amount of insulin. The adjusted insulin regimen for the flight is then calculated. Nonetheless, blood sugar should be checked often in order to counteract hyper- or hypoglycaemia.

5.11.2 Other metabolic disorders

In comparison to diabetes mellitus, with its time-critical medication and relatively exact dietary requirements, the other metabolic disorders remain in the backround. The patients are generally very well informed regarding the foods to be avoided. Of course, they may partake of the *airline's special catering.* They may also forego this and choose those items from the regular meal offering that are digestible and avoid the others. Certainly not all components are easy to discern regarding their composition, especially on return flights from Asia, given the different spices and dietary habits.

Often overlooked are such things as food colouring, preservatives, spice mixtures and flavour enhancers. Not all countries have such strict food regulations as Germany. Persons with known intolerances or *tendencies toward allergic reactions to foods* should utilize the *Special Meal* service to avoid unpleasant surprises.

Along these lines, a similar suggestion should be made regarding *snacks* such as peanuts, macadamia nuts, chips, or Asian rice pastries. People with predisposition should exercise caution and avoid the complimentary snack.

5.12 Surgeries

Preface

The evaluation of flight fitness following surgery is not a daily occurrence. In general, this is more likely to occur in a foreign country, but can also happen in Germany with ill patients who have had operations prior to their return flights. In that the indications for surgery almost always are related to acute situations rather than planned or elective procedures, these cases usually have complications relevant to aviation medicine. The type of operation also plays an important role, such as conventional or conservative surgical techniques in addition to the diagnosis, age of the patient, possible accompanying illnesses, or postoperative sequelae such as a colostomy.

In general, it can be assumed that *endoscopic procedures,* by virtue of their earlier symptom resolution, naturally heighten the patient's desire for a return flight! Here it is particularly important to make sure that the majority of the *filling gas in the abdomen* is resorbed in order to avoid uncomfortable symptoms due to the effect of gas expansion.

> The general recommendations given previously remain valid regarding flight fitness in commercial aircraft! Secondary transportation in an air ambulance can be performed under other criteria and can therefore take place much earlier than the cases discussed in the following.

5.12.1 Abdominal surgeries

The most common representatives besides appendectomies are cholecystectomies and urinary tract surgeries to remove kidney stones. Colon resections with or without reanastomosis are less common. The latter usually involves a primary disease such as a tumor and, due to additional medical aspects, makes evaluation more difficult.

In uncomplicated cases, such as **appendectomy without peritonitis** prior to perforation, an older patient may consider travel after 10 days, a younger after five, with respect to adequate wound healing. Infectious complications with delayed wound healing require at least three additional weeks. It is most important to take into consideration *Boyle-Mariottes gas law.* Because of the *expansion of bowel gas,* there is an increased stress on the wound and in the event of a rapid decompression wound dehiscence may occur. Among others, disrupted intestinal motility with local gas collection may result in symptoms similar to an ileus.

Cholecystectomy or **urinary tract surgeries** can result in earlier flight fitness disposition. Dependent upon the well-being of the patient, this may be the case after eight to ten days. But complications such as gall bladder peritonitis, among others, may extend this interval to 21 days or more.

The disposition of conventional **herniorrhaphies** (inguinal or umbilical) may be similar. After only five to eight days, if the general condition allows, and if the intervention was not endoscopic (resorption of filling gas!), the aeromedical disposition may be favourable.

Partial resection of the bowel is usually performed to treat stenotic lesions or tumors. Whether or not a colostomy is performed is of less importance. In every case, an invasion of the intestines with or without an interruption of continuity significantly affects function and especially motility. Again, the significance of the *Boyle-Mariotte law* with its effects must be emphasized. Secondly, the general medical condition with its accompanying medical problems is of particular importance! In these cases, a four-week postoperative interval before evaluation of flight fitness seems adequate. In specific cases fitness to fly can be evaluated earlier.

5.12.2 Neurosurgery

Previous neurosurgery that occurred a longer time ago carries no limitations per se. Of importance are the consequential complications or disabilities that may require an assistant.

Repatriation after a recent neurological intervention presents specific challenges. There is only one situation that arises repeatedly: an injury in a foreign country resulting in a *closed head injury* with subsequent neurological intervention and needing immediate *repatriation*.

Depending on the condition of the patient, transport may be carried out either *on a stretcher or in a* PTC.

Alert, oriented patients with spontaneous respirations are well managed on a stretcher. *Continence* is an important prerequisite. In uncertain cases, a urinary catheter and bowel preparation several days prior is indicated.

Other cases can only be transported by commercial airline if entirely separated from the rest of the cabin in a PTC *under intensive care conditions* with all other measures necessary for care provided.

> The environment of the modern commercial aircraft cabin is hypoxic and has the tendency to foster oedema!

It is well known that patients with such predispostion may develop early symptoms of high altitude sickness at pressures corresponding to 2,000 m. It cannot be known *when* and *how* this may occur on a flight, particularly when it involves a passenger weakened by illness. In order to *prevent hypoxia*, every case should have continuous supplemental oxygen provided with a flow of at least 4 l/min continuously. This flow is delivered at the switch position 0,9 of the Wenoll-System. *Medications for treatment of cerebral oedema* should be readily available and the patient must have sufficient *intravenous access* available in every case.

Decompression surgery such as for subdural haematomas or bleeding aneurysms are ready for transport relatively quickly after about two weeks if there are no other complicating conditions. It is important, even with normal circulatory parameters, satisfactory pulmonary function, and normal blood tests, to deliver continuous oxygen at a constant flow of 4 l/min (via Wenol system, 0.9 l/min on demand).

> Existence on intracranial, trapped air must have been ruled out!

5.12.3 Cardiopulmonary surgery

With regard to **cardiac surgery**, the primary disease is the main consideration. Reconstruction of congenital heart or valve replacement are not aeromedical concerns as the postoperative result is normal, or at least much improved. Even multiple bypass operations do not normally lead to any limitations after recovery. In the past it was common that passengers with CAD and bypass surgeries in foreign countries returned after a few days without any substantial complications.

With regard to **pulmonary surgeries**, once again, it is the primary disease that is the main consideration. Following resection of emphysematous bullae or surgical treatment of a pneumothorax, which may require a draining chest tube, a favourable disposition is usually possible. Pulmonary function has improved in the meantime. As long as the previously discussed requirements are met (see Preface, p. 114), a postoperative interval of one to two weeks is adequate in most cases.

For lobar resection, particular attention must be given to the underlying reason(s), such as tumors or tuberculosis. In these cases, adequate time for convalescence must be given in order to allow the rest of the lung to adapt to the new space.

5.13 Dental disorders

Preface

Dental treatments of any kind should be undertaken well in advance of a trip in order to make sure that the healing process is completed and there are no further complications such as bleeding or infection to be expected. In the event that a problem emerges during a flight, this may not necessarily affect the safety of the flight but would certainly affect the passenger's quality of life. At least three to four weeks should pass after *extractions, root canal treatment, or dental implants* prior to flight. This should not be a problem when planning a trip, as these procedures are usually elective.

5.13.1 Barodontalgia

Acute diseases of the oral cavity are rather uncommon and neglected aeromedical conditions. Nonetheless, many articles regarding this topic point out that they should not be underestimated. Additionally, incorrect pathophysiological processes are often attributed as causes. Still, inadequate dental restorations such as crowns, inlays or fillings are made out to be the culprits. The enclosed gas pockets allegedly expand in the reduced ambient pressure and supposedly cause pain. This theory has been proven wrong by numerous studies in hypobaric chambers with volunteer subjects with a defined cavity prepared in a dental filling.

Other mechanisms cause these unusual occurrences of barodontalgia in commercial airplanes. They must be evaluated not only with respect to aviation medicine, but particularly to general travel medicine.

Usually one finds dental root- and appliance-related infections which, under normal circumstances, do not cause discomfort and therefore are not discovered and treated. These infections often contain small, enclosed gas pockets, which do not have the ability to dissipate or be resorbed in the setting of inflammation. These gas pockets are subject to the *Boyle-Mariotte law*. They have no room to expand and therefore exert local pressure. This can press on the pulp and lead to pain. Nonetheless, the pressure differences found in commercial aviation are not so great as to be clinically relevant! This means that although the toothache is quite annoying, *in no case does it require an unplanned landing* for medical reasons.

! Since 2000, there have been no flight reports with acute dental problems!

There are other reasons why *dental examinations prior to flight* are a good idea! Every trip is stressful on the human body. In addition to the usual preparations and the ride to the airport, the vacation destination should be kept in mind. Other climates or dietary habits, such as spicy foods which are common in many tropical countries, can lead to a massive exacerbation of an otherwise harmless inflammation.

> To avoid a visit to a dentist during a vacation, with all the consequences such as language barriers, quality of treatment, financial problems, and a potentially ruined holiday, an appointment with your dentist prior to travel is strongly encouraged!

5.13.2 Implants

Regarding implants, numerous studies have shown that the pressure differential *does not lead to complications* even if the procedure was performed relatively recently. There is no increased risk of infection by invasion of bacteria. All experiments have resulted in sterile blood cultures. Problems can arise secondary to infection or trauma having occurred while at the vacation site.

6 Pregnancy and flight fitness

A normal pregnancy does not, of course, constitute an illness. Nonetheless, it is categorized by the Board of Medical Directors of IATA as a medical condition with the objective to avoid a medical event (emergency) on board.

> An uncomplicated pregnancy up to four weeks before the due date does not require any particular clearance for flight!

Radiation exposure in early pregnancy

Often the question is raised regarding flight during early pregnancy (first trimester) with respect to the consequences of *extraterrestrial radiation*. There is little information about this. Radiation typically involves two different conditions. On the one hand, it increases with altitude, as the protective effect of the atmosphere and magnetosphere decreases. On the other hand, the intensity is also dependent on geographic latitude. It increases up to 52° north and south, beyond which the value remains relatively constant. In the direction of the equator, activity is significantly reduced. In addition to a-, b-, and g-radiation, the so-called *solar flares* need to be considered; they have an 11-year cycle dependent on solar activity and are characterized by unpredictable and extremely strong activity. An average flight from Europe to the west coast of the USA entails about 30 µSv, a flight to Rio de Janeiro only results in 18 µSv, while the strongest exposure of 62 µSv has been measured on flights to Japan via the polar route.

> **!** Thus, there are a number of reasons to avoid flying during early pregnancy.

As in all other cases, there are concerns of increased infection, climate-induced circulatory problems, and travel stress.

Flight close to date of delivery?

During the last four weeks of pregnancy flying is possible from a medical point of view, but it is prudent for the treating obstetrician to consult with the Lufthansa physician or aviation medicine specialist of the particular airline in order to rule out any contraindications.

On-board births occur very rarely. Since 1956 only 15 deliveries have been reported.

7 Travelling with children (medical advice)

Travelling with children – especially young children – is particularly challenging for parents. It should be evaluated repeatedly and carefully whether the vacation destination with all its local conditions as well as the journey itself are appropriate for (young) children or babies.

Regarding the trip to the airport, one should take advantage of the possibility to *check in on the evening before*, especially with charter flights which often are scheduled early in the morning. The disadvantage of an additional overnight stay is far outweighed by stress-free boarding without luggage. One must always be aware of the current security regulations!

The medical recommendations for children naturally are the same as those for adults. There are additional recommendations to avoid stressful situations:

1. Each child should have its own *age-appropriate hand luggage*. This should include a favorite toy and a variety of items to pass the time such as books, drawing materials, music, story cassettes or an electronic toy. One should make sure that there is an adequate supply of batteries.
2. Additionally, parents should be ready to engage in individual activities with the children and be prepared to pass the time with *games, puzzles, or guessing games* during long flights or delays.

3. *Snacks* are important for children on long flights, as they are also activities and play a role in passing the time. Although there is a limit to the amount of drinks one can bring (100 ml per container), baby food and snacks are only permitted with a medical letter and bottles of *baby food must be opened at the security check point*. This means that there is a risk of contamination and it may lead to intestinal problems or even illness. Since the schedule for meal service on board is quite rigid, it is advisable to purchase food after passing through security.

A tip for food storage

The temperature in the luggage storage areas over the seats is much lower than in the cabin, and is similar to refrigerators. Therefore there is little danger of food spoilage.

8   Travelling with toddlers (legal regulations)

Toddlers are defined as children who have not yet reached their second birthday.

There are significant restrictions for these children on board of commercial airplanes in order to ensure they travel safe and comfortable.

The number of travelling children is limited by:

1. The number of rows of seats in the cabin (One toddler per row is the maximum allowed. Exceptions are rows with child seats. Here, the number of toddlers is limited by the number of child seats available)
2. The availability of child seats
3. The number of personal floatation devices for toddlers on board

On intercontinental flights, the number of toddlers normally is restricted to 15.

On continental flights, the number of toddlers travelling is limited by the number of seat rows excluding those that are emergency exit rows. On *flights over water* more than 50 nautical miles (about 94 km) from the coast, the limit is 10 toddlers.

9 Disabled passengers

Passengers with disabilities or limited mobility can request the assistance needed on the ground as well as on board when making their reservations.

In individual cases, it may be necessary for the treating physician to fill out the MEDIF (Medical Information Form) which can be obtained from the reservations department, to ensure that the required support is provided. The forms are available in paper and electronic versions.

The MEDIF and the FREMEC (Frequent Traveller's Medical Card) are issued by Lufthansa's medical department. The blank forms contain the necessary conditions and information regarding care during flight.

For non-ambulatory or paralyzed passengers, wheelchairs are available at airports at no extra cost if they are not travelling with their own personal wheelchair.

When making the reservation one should indicate whether a personal wheelchair will be used for the trip or arrangements should be made for a wheelchair to be available at the departure and/or destination airport. If a personal wheelchair is used, its dimensions and weight as well as special functions (collapsible/not collapsible, sport wheelchair, etc.) must be disclosed.

If a personal wheelchair is taken along on the flight, there will not be any additional charges to transport it, but it must be checked into the cargo hold as it cannot be used on board due to the narrow aisles.

If a passenger wants to travel with a *battery-operated wheelchair*, he or she must be knowledgeable about the type of battery and provide this information when booking the flight. Gel, dry, or sealed wet batteries may stay on the wheelchair. At check-in, they must be secured and disconnected, and the leads must be isolated from each other. Non-sealed batteries cannot be transported due to safety reasons.

A special on-board wheelchair is provided on Lufthansa's long-haul flights. This is a collapsible wheelchair with special functions that can operate without problems in the narrow aisles due to its slim shape and transport handicapped passengers to and from their seats. Some of the rest rooms on board the long-haul airplanes are a bit more spacious, allowing the disabled passenger to use the facility without assistance.

Blind or deaf passengers are accepted on all Lufthansa flights. They must be offered any and all necessary assistance by the airline representatives in order to assure a safe and comfortable flight. They have the option to take along a *guide dog* at no extra cost but the number of animals allowed in the cabin is limited. The regulations with respect to bringing animals to foreign countries must also be considered. The dog should be muzzled while in the cabin.

9.1 The MEDIF/MEDA forms

In order to communicate with ill passengers, their treating physicians, and the airline personnel helping to arrange the patient transport, the *Medical Information Form (MEDIF) – sometimes called Medical Data Advice (MEDA)* form – is essential. These forms are available from the travel agencies through which the flights were booked, or directly from airline. It is an usually IATA-standardized form.

Patient clarification and the resulting flight approval for ill passengers are accepted by all IATA airlines if an authorized physician of an IATA airline gives the so-called *Doc OK* on the MEDIF/MEDA form. Thus, codeshare flights (flights within a network of cooperating airlines) or flights via multiple connections with a variety of IATA airlines are normally not a problem for the medically evaluated and approved passenger.

The MEDIF form (see Fig. 27 and 28 on the subsequent pages) is required for passengers
- with skull or brain injuries or internal or significant external injuries (wounds, burns)

Deutsche Lufthansa AG | Passenger Medical Care FRA PM/C | Frankfurt am Main, Germany

Information Sheet for Passengers Requiring Special Assistance – Special Assistance Form

⊘ **Lufthansa**

In accordance with IATA Resolution 700 Attachment A, 29th Edition, June 2009

1.
Name, first name	Title	Age	Gender

2.
Passenger Name Record (PNR) / Amadeus filekey (FK)			

3.
Routing from	to	Flight number	Class	Date

4. Type of disability or required assistance

5. Stretcher transport required ☐ Yes ☐ No
☐ STCR Must travel on a stretcher. This requires medical assistance, either nurse/paramedic or a physician.
☐ PTC Intercont intensive care services available on specific A/C. MOC assists with clearance and booking.

6. Escort for the journey required ☐ Yes ☐ No
Designated escort (Name)   Medical qualification
☐ physician ☐ nurse/paramedic ☐ none
☐ other applicable person (Name)   PNR (if different)

7. Wheelchair required ☐ Yes ☐ No
☐ WCHR Ambulant but impaired in walking: Needs assistance in terminal to/from gate, needs wheelchair or similar when passengers are boarded/disembarking by walking over ramp. Does not need assistance in a ramp bus, on passenger steps and in the aircraft cabin to/from seat, toilets and with meals.

☐ WCHS Ambulant but more severely limited in walking: Cannot use a ramp bus and needs assistance in boarding/disembarking (e.g. on passenger steps). Does not need assistance in the aircraft cabin to/from seat, toilets and with meals.

☐ WCHC Non-ambulant: Needs also assistance in the aircraft to/from seat, toilets and possibly with meals

Own wheelchair Battery-driven collapsible Size (W/H/L cm) Weight (kg)
☐ WCH OWN ☐ WCH BD / dry batteries ☐

8. Hospital at destination ☐ Yes ☐ No
Designated Ambulance (to be organized by assistance/insurance/passenger)
contact (phone/email)

9. Assistance/support while in the airport required ☐ Yes ☐ No
Designated person/organisation
contact (phone/email)

10. Other assistance/support while in the airport required ☐ Yes ☐ No
Which and where? Departure/transit/arrival? Organized by assistance/insurance/passenger
contact (phone/email)

11. Specific needs/support/equipment required in-flight/on board ☐ Yes ☐ No
Please specify (e.g. special meal, extra seat, type of equipment, etc.)

Facultative expenses on account of passenger. **For oxygen concentrator please ask for the specific document.**
Technical clearance issued by airline ☐ Yes ☐ No
FREMEC (Frequent Medical Traveller Card) ☐ Yes ☐ No
12. Valid until   Issued by

The conditions of carriage, in particular the rules of liability contained in the terms and conditions of Lufthansa German Airline, will apply.

Contact: Medical Operation Center (MOC) | Phone: +49 69 696 55077 | Lufthansa AG
email: medicaloperation@dlh.de | Fax: ++49 69 696 83677 | Frankfurt am Main, Germany

Fig. 27 MEDIF form, page 1

Deutsche Lufthansa AG | Passenger Medical Care FRA PM/C | Frankfurt am Main, Germany

Information Sheet for Passengers Requiring Medical Clearance – MEDIF Part 1

In accordance with IATA Resolution 700 Attachment B, 29th Edition, June 2009

Note for the attending physician:

The details requested in here will be treated confidentially; they should enable the Medical Services of the airline(s), as it is their obligation, to judge by their specific air medical knowledge and experience if and under what conditions the patient can be permitted to travel by aircraft as requested. These details will also help the Medical Service in issuing appropriate instructions for the patient's care which duly consider both his/her diagnosis and the special circumstances of the requested air journey.

Kindly answer all questions by cross or in block letters, as necessary. Please fill in this form on your PC to enhance readability and clarity. You can easily typewrite into the grey fields. Thank you for your cooperation!

For any further information please do not hesitate to contact us immediately via phone or email.

1.	**Patient's name**			
	Date of Birth	Sex	Height	Weight
2.	**Attending physician**			
	Address			
	e-mail	Telephone, indicate country and area code		Fax

3. **Diagnosis** (including short history, onset of current illness, episode or accident and treatment, specify if contagious)

Nature and date of any recent and/or relevant surgery

4. **Current symptoms and severity**   **Date of onset**

5. **Will a 25% to 30% reduction in the ambient partial pressure of oxygen (relative hypoxia) affect the passenger's medical condition?** (Cabin pressure to be the equivalent of a fast trip to a mountain elevation of 2.400 meters (8.000 feet) above sea level) ☐ yes ☐ no ☐ not sure

6. **Additional clinical information** ☐ yes ☐ no

    a. Anemia ☐ yes ☐ no

        If yes, give recent result in grams of haemoglobin per litre

    b. Psychiatric conditions ☐ yes ☐ no If yes, see Part 2

    c. Cardiac disorder ☐ yes ☐ no If yes, see Part 2

    d. Normal bladder control ☐ yes ☐ no If no, give mode of control

    e. Normal bowel control ☐ yes ☐ no

    f. Respiratory disorder ☐ yes ☐ no If yes, see Part 2

    g. Does the patient require oxygen at home? ☐ yes ☐ no If yes, specify how much

    h. Oxygen needed during flight? ☐ yes ☐ no If yes, specify ☐ 2 LPM ☐ 4 LPM other

    i. Seizure disorder ☐ yes ☐ no If yes, see Part 2

7. **Escort**

    a. Is the patient fit to travel unaccompanied? ☐ yes ☐ no

    b. Is the patient able to sit in a usual aircraft seat? ☐ yes ☐ no

    c. Is the patient able to embark and disembark the aircraft independently? ☐ yes ☐ no

    d. If no, will the patient have a private escort to take care of his/her needs onboard? ☐ yes ☐ no

    e. If yes, who should escort the passenger? ☐ Doctor ☐ Nurse/Paramedic ☐ Other

    f. If other, is the escort fully capable to attend to all above needs? ☐ yes ☐ no

8. **Mobility**

    a. able to walk without assistance ☐ yes ☐ no b. Wheelchair required for boarding ☐ to aircraft ☐ to seat

9. **Medication list** (incl. doses)

10. **Other medical information**

Contact: Medical Operation Center (MOC) | Phone: +49 69 696 55077 | Lufthansa AG
email: medicaloperation@dlh.de | Fax: ++49 69 696 83677 | Frankfurt am Main, Germany

Fig. 28a MEDIF part 1

Deutsche Lufthansa AG   Passenger Medical Care FRA PM/C   Frankfurt am Main, Germany

Information Sheet for Passengers Requiring Medical Clearance – MEDIF Part 2

⊘ **Lufthansa**

In accordance with IATA Resolution 700 Attachment B, 29th Edition, June 2009

1. Cardiac condition

  a. Angina   ☐ yes ☐ no   When was last episode?

    - Is the condition stable?   ☐ yes ☐ no

    - Functional class of the patient?   ☐ No symptoms   ☐ Angina with moderate exertion

       ☐ Angina with minimal exertion   ☐ Angina at rest

    - Can the patient walk 100 metres at a normal pace or climb 10-12 stairs without symptoms? ☐ yes ☐ no

  b. Myocardial infarction   ☐ yes ☐ no   Date

    - Complications?   ☐ yes ☐ no   If yes, give details

    - Stress EKG done?   ☐ yes ☐ no   If yes, what was the result?   MET or   Watt

    - If angioplasty or coronary bypass,

       can patient walk 100 yards/metres at a normal pace or climb 10-12 stairs without symptoms? ☐ yes ☐ no

  c. Cardiac failure   ☐ yes ☐ no   When was last episode?

    - Is the patient controlled with medication?   ☐ yes ☐ no

    - Functional class of the patient?   ☐ No symptoms ☐ Shortness of breath (SOB) with moderate exertion

       ☐ SOB with minimal exertion   ☐ Shortness of breath at rest

  d. Syncope   ☐ yes ☐ no   When was last episode?

    - Investigations   ☐ yes ☐ no   If yes, state results

2. Chronic pulmonary condition   ☐ yes ☐ no

  a. Has the patient had recent arterial blood gases?   ☐ yes ☐ no

  b. Blood gases were taken on   ☐ room air   ☐ Oxygen   litres per minute (LPM)

     If yes, what were the results pCO_2 [kPa/mmHg] pO_2 [kPa/mmHg]

       % Saturation   Date of exam

  c. Does the patient retain CO_2?   ☐ yes ☐ no

  d. Has his/her condition deteriorated recently?   ☐ yes ☐ no

  e. Can patient walk 100 yards/metres at a normal pace or climb 10-12 stairs without symptoms? ☐ yes ☐ no

  f. Has the patient ever taken a commercial aircraft in in his/her current medical status?   ☐ yes ☐ no

    - If yes, when?

    - Did the patient have any problems?

3. Psychiatric conditions   ☐ yes ☐ no

  a. Is there a possibility that the patient will become agitated during flight?   ☐ yes ☐ no

  b. Has he/she taken a commercial aircraft before?   ☐ yes ☐ no

    - If yes, date of travel?   Did the patient travel   ☐ alone   ☐ escorted?

4. Seizure   ☐ yes ☐ no

  a. What type of seizures?

  b. Frequency of the seizures

  c. When was the last seizure?

  d. Are the seizures controlled by medication?   ☐ yes ☐ no

5. Prognosis for the trip   ☐ Good   ☐ Poor

Physician signature (or facsimile) _____   Date

Note: Cabin attendants are not authorized to give special assistance (e.g. lifting, feeding) to particular passengers, to the detriment of their service to other passengers. Additionally, they are trained only in **first aid** and are not permitted to administer any injection, or give medication. **Important:** Fees, if any, relevant to the provision of the above information and for carrier-provided special equipment are to be paid by the passenger concerned.

Contact: Medical Operation Center (MOC)   Phone: +49 69 696 55077   Lufthansa AG
email: medicaloperation@dlh.de   Fax: ++49 69 696 83677   Frankfurt am Main, Germany

Fig. 28 b MEDIF part 2

- with multiple sclerosis
- with spastic paralysis with psychological handicaps
- with mental disorders
- for passengers who wish to fly within six months after a heart attack or three months after a stroke
- who require special devices during flight (oxygen, breathing equipment, incubator, infusions, etc.)
- who cannot travel in a non-reclined airline seat (necessitating a stretcher)

This form is being adopted and standardized by all IATA airlines.

The treating physician fills out the page *Medical Information By Attending Physician*, disclosing the details regarding diagnosis, illness, and prognosis for the trip and answering various questions that are crucial for assessing the patient's flight fitness and/or the necessary assistance on the ground and on board.

The first page of the MEDIF form (see Fig. 27) is needed to identify the flight routes and the necessary preparations for the flight booked by an ill or mobility-limited passenger. If no special medical clarification or clearance is required, only Section 1 of the form needs to be filled out. It should be provided to the travel agency as soon as possible in order to prepare for the necessary arrangements, such as a stretcher, supplemental oxygen, or wheelchair, in time for the intended flight.

The second page of the MEDIF form (see Fig. 28) must always be filled out if clarification of the passenger's medical condition by an authorized airline physician is required. All medical information on this page is kept strictly private and follows the rules of medical confidentiality in Germany according to Sect. 203 StGB. They are revealed only to the airline's authorized physician to determine flight fitness and to confirm or modify the requested special arrangements for the flight. Page 2 of the MEDIF form is also filled out by the treating physician. It is very important that handwritten entries are legible. The medical information should be precise, reflect the actual situation, and be detailed enough that the evaluating airline physician can obtain a clear basis for a determination.

On the page Handling Advice Invalid Passenger the airline physician or contract physician documents the decision for the airline, under what circumstances the patient is fit to fly (assistant, possible pre- and post-flight transportation with an ambulance, oxygen), and determines the necessary support:

- **ESCORT**: Passenger must be accompanied (if yes, e.g. by a physician or other appropriate person)
- **WCH**: Wheelchair passenger
- **WCHR** (**R** for ramp): Able to walk, but with impaired mobility
  - Requires assistance in the terminal to/from the gate, and wheelchair or other assistance when boarding/deplaning requires walking on apron

- Does not require assistance on the airport bus, on the aircraft stairway, in the cabin to the seat or restrooms, or with meals
- **WCHS** (**S** for steps): Able to walk, but significantly disabled
  - Cannot use an airport bus and needs assistance to board and deplane (e.g. via aircraft stairway)
  - Does not require assistance in the cabin (to and from the seat or restrooms, or with meals)
- **WCHS/OWN**: As above – brings own wheelchair along (add **BD** if battery-operated wheelchair)
- **WCHC** (**C** for cabin): Not ambulatory
  - Needs assistance in the cabin to and from the seat and restrooms, and possibly with meals (provide necessary details)
- **BED**: Requires a stretcher
- **AMBULANCE**: Requires an ambulance at the destination, ordered by the airline and charged to the patient
- **OXYGEN OCCASIONAL/CONTINUOUS**: Requires occasional or continuous oxygen during flight
- **BLND**: Blind or severely visually impaired passenger
- **DEAF**: Deaf passenger
- Other required support/measures (on the ground, during flight) and/or provisions arranged by the physician
- **FREMEC** issued by the airline

9.2 The Frequent Traveller's Medical Card

The FREMEC can be issued to patients with chronic medical conditions or permanent disabilities on the basis of the information disclosed in the MEDIF if they travel frequently. The *Frequent Traveller's Medical Card* contains all the documentation needed for care and replaces the MEDIF otherwise required for each flight (see Fig. 29 and 30). The expiration date is dependent on the medical situation.

The individual service packet is determined according to the information on the FREMEC. If, for example, the abbreviation WCHC is noted on the FREMEC, the airline personnel will know that this is a passenger who can neither walk nor stand. In this case, a caretaker is required to order to assist the passenger from his or her own wheelchair into the one supplied at the airport.

A valid FREMEC must be presented at each booking to allow designation of the required assistance without renewed medical clarification, as long as the health status has not changed.

It is recommended that a copy of the FREMEC pass be kept in a safe place so that in can be duplicated without difficulty if lost.

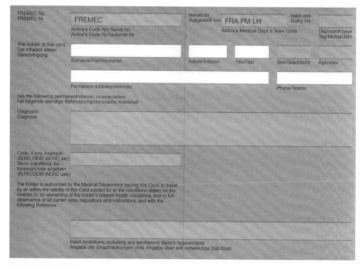

Conditions of Issue

1.
Cardholders are required to report all changes in their present handicap or incapacitation and/or the deterioration in their physical or medical condition, to the airline representative or agent with whom they are in contact.

2.
Subject to all terms and conditions on this card, the authorisation for air travel is valid only up to the date stated on the front.

3.
This card is not transferable and must be produced, together with proof of the cardholder's identity, on every occasion whenever airline reservations are made for the cardholder, at time of ticket issuance, and when so requested by the airlines or their agents or representatives.

4.
Cardholders are reminded that arrangements for travel should be made as much in advance as possible. They should also allow sufficient time for check-in formalities.

1.
Der Ausweis-Inhaber ist verpflichtet, alle Veränderungen des gegenwärtigen Zustandes seiner Behinderung/Krankheit, und/oder die Verschlechterung seines Gesundheitszustandes, der Luftverkehrsgesellschaft (oder Reisebüro), bei der (dem) eine Buchung vorgenommen wird, mitzuteilen.

2.
Diese Genehmigung hat unter den genannten Bedingungen nur bis zu dem umseitig genannten Datum Gültigkeit.

3.
Diese Genehmigung ist nicht übertragbar. Sie muß, unter Legitimation des Inhabers, bei der Buchung eines Fluges, Ausstellung eines Flugscheines und wann immer Einschränkung gefordert wird, der Luftverkehrsgesellschaft, dem Reisebüro oder dem Beauftragten vorgelegt werden.

4.
Der Ausweis-Inhaber wird gebeten, die Reisevorbereitungen möglichst früh vor Reiseantritt zu treffen und am Abreisetag genügend Zeit für die Fluggast-abfertigung einzuplanen.

Form 8704 A-00 (FRA PM) Printed in the Federal Republic of Germany

Frequent Traveller's Medical Card
Ärztlicher Ausweis für Fluggäste (FREMEC)

Lufthansa

The data contained in the shaded fields must always be transmitted with any reservation request.

Die Angaben in den gerasterten Feldern sind in jeder Buchungsanfrage zu übermitteln.

Date and Place of Issue
Datum/Ort der Ausstellung

Passenger's Signature
(Legal guardian or Passenger's witness may sign if passenger is physically unable to do so).
Unterschrift des Fluggastes
(oder Unterschrift des gesetzlichen Vertreters)

Fig. 29   FREMEC, cover

Fig. 30   FREMEC, inside

9.3 Disabled passengers and passengers with reduced mobility

Regarding unaccompanied disabled passengers, the regulations of the *Luftfahrt-Bundesamt*, LBA (Federal office of civil aviation), must be observed!

In the past as well as today air travel for disabled passengers or people with reduced mobility have always caused a lot of organisational problems. While at least in Europe in the past a disabled passenger was considered as somebody ill and requiring medical care and thus subject to IATA travel regulations for the sick, meanwhile there have been significant changes. A disabled passenger is no longer to be considered ill but a person with certain restrictions in his daily life. Therefore the IATA guidelines are no longer fully applicable in their existing form. Another important point is the fact that these regulations are only advisory but not obligatory.

Nevertheless, the national laws of the state where the plane is registered, the so-called *Flag Right* (see Chapter I.8.2 and I.8.3) applies. The national aviation authorities, i.e. the *Luftfahrtbundesamt* in Germany or the *Federal Aviation Agency* in the United States have established safety based standards, which may impose certain restrictions on the group of passengers in question.

Already several years ago the United States started to clearly distinguish between *disabled* and *ill* persons. This is reflected in the relevant legislation.

A disabled person is defined as somebody suffering from temporary or permanent physical or mental limitations. That does not only cover for the limitations mentioned above but even for drug- or alcohol dependancy!

This is quite different from European legislation, which has to be incorporated into national legislation. The correspondent texts are to be found in 49 U.S.C. § 41705 a resp. EU-OPS EC 1107/2006.

This means that new obligations will be imposed upon the airlines, which to a certain extent also have implications on the airports. Nevertheless, in the final analysis it is always the airline which is responsible, even if airports have been remiss!

But the handicapped person or PRM (passenger with reduced mobility) too must consider and follow certain rules when planning air travel. As mentioned before there are clearly defined differences between European and U.S. laws. While in the U.S. a disabled person has to report before the flight only if they are in need of special devices – as e.g. additional oxygen – but not for e.g. wheelchairs, in the European Union they have to communicate their special medical requirements at least 48 hours in advance.

There are major differences if MEDIF is required (see Chapter II.9.1 *The MEDIF/ MEDA forms*).

However, these forms only apply to ill passengers (in contrast to PRM), whether it is an acute state or chronic disease that may or may not interfere with air travel. In Europe the form must be completed in some cases – disorders or risks – that do not require reporting in the United States. The Airline may thus be in breach of American legislation and run the risk of being sued. It is of course the duty and obligation of the airports to implement these regulations in a practicable way. It is not the responsibility of the attending or consulting physician.

However, there is more transparency concerning the reasons, why in certain circumstances air travel may be impossible for disabled persons or PRMs or only possible with certain supportive measures.

This means then that in each case the medical and also the legal situation should be carefully evaluated to not only ensure comfortable conditions of travel for the person in question but also make sure that all the assistance required is also available at the airports.

The following synopsis will show the differences and similarities between the United States and the European Union.

Definition and Rights for Disabled or PRMs

DOT 14 C.F.R. Part 382	EU No. 1107/2006
Categories covered under Part 382 are individuals with permanent or temporary physical or mental impairment	Categories covered under EU 1107/2006 are all persons with reduced mobility when using air transport
Physical impairment, disorders or conditions visual, speech, hearing impairments, anatomical losses, musculoskeletal or cosmetic disfigurement, cardiovascular, digestive or metabolic disorders, epilepsy, cancer	**Any permanent/temporary physical disability** sensoral or locomotor, visual, speech, hearing impairments, passengers requiring a wheelchair to and from the aircraft in any form.
Mental or psychological disorders mental retardation, emotional or mental illness	**Intellectual disability or impairment** as in U.S. Part 382
Passengers using medical oxygen or respiratory devices	(No comparable comment)
Carriers must ensure that the provided services (boarding, deboarding, transit etc.) within the airports meet Part 382.	Airports are responsible to provide services within it's area.

DOT 14 C.F.R. Part 382	EU No. 1107/2006

Attention

Carriers may be held responsible if any european airport does not meet the requirements of Part 382. The carrier then must supplement such services!

Carriers cannot generally require passengers with a disabilty to provide advanced notice	Passengers should notice carriers at least 48 hours in advance

Attention

European airports might face major difficulties assisting a significant number of disabled passengers arriving, departing or transiting at the same time without advance notice!

Carriers cannot generally require passengers to have a medical certificate or undergo preflight medical clearance.	Passengers with medical conditions are not covered under EC 1107/2006.

Exceptions: stretcher, oxygen during flight, communicable disease posing direct threat, unable to complete the flight safely.	*Medical certificate or clearance may be requested* fitness to travel is in doubt, contagious disease, operation, potential hazard of diversion.

Attention

European carriers flying to/from the U.S. requesting a medical certificate if passenger's fitness to travel is doubtful may violate Part 382!

Passengers may be refused from transportation only for communicable diseases posing a direct threat to others! The condition must be both to be directly transmitted and having serious health consequences i.e. SARS, H1N1, Avian flu etc.	Carriers may request a *Fitness to fly* or refuse transportation.

Attention

European carriers flying to or from the U.S. refusing a passenger with Influenza A (H1N1) may violate Part 382!

Certification from manufacturer that FAA requirements are met: tested and meeting the RTCA conditions securly stowable battery operated.	**Not covered under EC 1107/2006** Assuming the device as dangerous good, EU-OPS states that carriers must not transport the device in the cabin.

Attention

Complete new regulation! Only a few if any devices are labelled meeting these FAA requirements! Additional approval mandatory to meet EU-OPS!

Air carriers must not limit the number of passengers with a disability on a scheduled flight.	EU-OPS recommends reducing the number of PRMs in order not to exceed the number of passengers able to assist in an emergency evacuation.

DOT 14 C.F.R. Part 382	EU No. 1107/2006

Attention

DOT does not accept a conflict of exception as EASA does by recommending a limited number. Limitation might become mandatory at the end of 2009.

Air carriers may require from a disabled or PRM to be accompanied by an attendant only for safety reasons. If a Safety Assistant is imposed contrary to the passenger's self assessment, the assistant travels for free.	Air carriers may require that a PRM or passenger with disabilities travels with another person which provides the requested assistance.
Air carriers must not refuse transportation to a passenger with a disability on the basis of his or her disability.	Air carriers may refuse transportation to meet applicable safety requirements established by ■ international law ■ community or national law ■ size of the aircraft or it's doors making boarding impossible
Foreign carriers will not be required to carry any service animals in the cabin except dogs. **Evidence must be accepted by a credible verbal assurance of the disabled or** ■ presence of harness, tags etc. ■ written official documentation ■ identification card	**Air carriers must only carry recognized assistance dogs in the cabin (subject to national regulation)** Assistant dogs are accepted and affiliated to the International Dog Fedaration and trained by an ADI approved organisation (Assistant Dogs International).
Carriers must make a *Complaint Resolution Official (CRO)* available at each destination the carrier serves (person or hotline) CROs must have the authority to resolve complaints definitely with the power to overrule other carrier personnel. CRO must answer the complainant in written form describing the correction action within a period of 30 days.	EU Member States have to create or nominate a *National Enforcement Body* for complaints of passengers feeling treated not correct. Acknowledgement of receipt must be given within 2 weeks. Case submission to the airline requiring a comment within 6 weeks from date of the receipt.

Requirements for an assistant

An assistant must be:

■ Physically capable to bring the handicapped person to the emergency exit and to assist with boarding and deboarding

■ Familiar with the particular needs of the handicapped individual during the entire flight (meals, use of restrooms, medications and assistance during flight anomalies)

III

Treatment of medical emergencies on board

1 Medical diversions

During the treatment of an on-board emergency, questions may arise in some cases whether a diversion for medical reasons should be performed.

According to which criteria should a captain be advised to divert?

Certainly this should always be determined by the treating physician, but there are other aspects pertaining to a variety of technical aeronautical issues that must be taken into consideration. The doctor's recommendation is not a mandatory order!

The following perspectives, among others, are to be taken into medical consideration:

- Condition of the patient
  (instability, further anticipated complications)
- Ability of the physician within his or her clinical specialty and the possible need for intervention (such as intubation, ventilation by mask)
- Equipment – what is available?
- Is assistance available? (such as necessary CPR)
- Urgent indication for immediate hospitalization (such as following successful resuscitation)

In addition, there are the aeronautical decision processes:

- Distance to the next suitable airport (runway length, size of apron, availability of tugs, etc.)
- Procedural requirements for the flight profile (such as high stairway for Airbus A380, fuelling requirements, external power/hydraulics/pressurization procedures)
- Weight of the aircraft, and the ability for *fuel dumping* (fuel is jettisoned to attain the allowed landing weight, which can take 30 minutes or more to accomplish!)
- Medical facilities available at the diversion site (ambulances, appropriate hospital facility, etc.)
- Regulatory requirements of the crew – will they exceed their time limit or can they continue their shift; if a replacement crew is needed, accommodating the passengers during a layover may be necessary (hotel availability?)

For these reasons, it may be more reasonable not to choose the nearest airport, but to utilize the time needed in any case to address the abovementioned operative aspects and fly a little further to approach a better suited and prepared destination. This also allows more time to plan for an immediate transfer of the patient to the receiving hospital.

The cockpit crew has access at all times to a database containing the relevant information regarding suitable airports along the route. Not only is there aeronautical information, but there is also extensive data on local hospitals, their current local contact information, bed capacity, diagnostic and therapeutic facilities, and ambulance capabilities.

Regarding the regulatory aspects of decision-making on board, please see Chapter I.8.1.

Death on board

Acute death or death occurring during treatment on board is a rare incident. A detailed review at *Lufthansa German Airlines AG* showed between 5 and 14 cases per year, which in relation to the previously reported passenger loads, is an extremely small proportion and is significantly below the average death rate of comparable groups. Nonetheless, particularly for these cases, the procedures are worth to mention. There are two different conceivable scenarios:

- A passenger is found dead in his or her seat, e.g. after a night flight or at the start of cabin service. After death has been ascertained, the body should be brought to the aft galley if possible, covered, and stored. To the extent possible, it should be wedged against the wall with blankets in order to avoid any slippage. In the Boeing B747, the upper deck galley is the natural choice. If the deceased person was seated in the front part of the aircraft, one would obviously utilize the forward area of the cabin.

■ If resuscitation has been unsuccessful, the previous procedure should be followed.

In any such case, *a diversion is not recommended*. The affected person cannot be helped any further, and an unplanned landing would only create problems with the relatives of the deceased and the other passengers: decontamination and quarantine regulations, undetermined causes of death with potential legal consequences and subsequent transport of the corpse back home.

Declaration of death is made by the attending physician, but he or she does not issue a *death certificate*. This is a matter for the health authorities at the destination airport, who can then initiate an autopsy.

> Lufthansa transports more than 75 million passengers annually. The medical department receives about 2,500–3,000 reports every year about medical incidents from the cabin crew. Life-threatening or fatal situations, fortunately, are quite rare. In more than 80% of cases, there is a physician among the passengers, who can then resort to the extensive medical equipment on board.

2   General considerations regarding medical emergencies

2.1   Assistance from flight attendants

Even though flight attendants in the early days of commercial aviation were trained nurses, these qualifications did not become a standard in the following decades.

Prior to employment at Lufthansa, flight attendants must pass a first aid course consisting of 16 hours. Building on this initial schooling, the knowledge base is further deepened during basic training, whereby the particulars of on-board assistance, the available medical equipment, and the standardized protocols are taught.

By regulation, flight attendants must take a four-hour refresher course in first aid every year, which focuses primarily on *cardiopulmonary resuscitation* and *AED training,* as well as practising the most common emergency situations.

The *purser* – or lead flight attendant – receives additional medical training to be able to coordinate the medical assistance procedure.

In general, one can expect flight attendants to have a *good understanding of first aid under the special circumstances on board*. They cannot, however, be expected to act as fully-fledged medical assistants to the attending physician, as the low incidence of emergency situations on board does not provide the necessary experience and confidence regarding use of the equipment.

2.2 Decision-making for cardiopulmonary resuscitation

Flight attendants are required to begin life-saving measures immediately and to continue CPR until the patient has either regained consciousness or has been turned over to medical personnel on the ground.

In addition to CPR, they may not take any further therapeutic measures other than the application of the AED and oxygen.

Additional medical emergency equipment may, as a rule, only be used by physicians or other qualified medical technicians. Exceptions are only allowed by permission of the captain.

In individual cases, the captain can decide whether an other appropriately trained person may overstep legal limitations to use medications or equipment in an emergency to save the patient's life.

2.3 Diagnostic and therapeutic options

Emergency medical equipment makes it possible for the assisting physician to take a history and to perform a symptom-based examination. In many cases, the physician can identify the suspected medical condition or at least properly assess the possible threats to the patient.

To verify a suspected diagnosis, the *diagnostic tools* available to the physician include:

- Blood pressure measurement
- Temperature measurement with a strip thermometer
- Blood glucose measurement with an electronic device
- Measurement of oxygen saturation with a finger pulse oximeter

The physician's mere presence, positive assessment of the situation and judicious use of medication will already ameliorate the symptoms in many cases.

Should the condition of the patient not improve or at least stabilize, a diversion may be considered after consultation with the crew.

The final decision is made by the captain!

2.4 Space limitations

In-seat examination and treatment of the patient is generally limited to the less complicated and unambiguous medical conditions.

Otherwise, the patient should be brought to the *galley* where curtains can provide additional privacy and the patient, as well as the assistants, can be blocked from the view of other passengers. Here it is also possible to perform a more detailed examination, to lay out the emergency equipment, or in case of deterioration, to initiate resuscitation without delay.

2.5 Illumination

Especially during night flights, the darkened cabin makes it difficult to perform an examination without disturbing the other passengers. Here one must either evaluate the patient at his or her seat with one of the many *flashlights* on board or bring the patient to the galley in order to have better lighting.

In acute situations, the *cabin lights* would be turned on to render better care or to find a qualified assistant if one did not identify him- or herself after the initial announcement.

2.6 Noise

Even though the *stethoscope* is a necessary part of diagnostic medical equipment, it is of *limited value* on board.

Useful auscultatory findings regarding the heart, lungs or abdomen are the exception.

The surrounding noise, primarily from the engines and the air conditioning system, make it difficult to obtain a blood pressure measurement by auscultation. It is therefore helpful to obtain the systolic pressure by palpation at the wrist.

3 Motion sickness

Also known as travel sickness, or sea- or airsickness, these symptom complexes are grouped together as motion sickness as they generally occur in humans in response to passive movement in space.

Our original socialization with regard to movement patterns (speed of walking, limited acceleration and deceleration effects, upright head and body position, limited multidimensional components, predominantly self-controlled body movements, preservation of optical control) continues regardless, and is dependent on individual differences and existing environmental conditions.

> Due to genetic predisposition, about 10% of people are immune against the development of motion sickness while another 10% are very susceptible. The rest lies somewhere in between.

Children under two years are practically immune, as "rolling" movements are rather calming and induce sleep. Older children can undergo a type of optical-kinetic learning process through to the end of puberty which can lead to a certain motion sickness resistance in adulthood. This is somewhat more pronounced in males.

Although a large number of passengers on ships in turbulent seas develop significant symptoms, only *relatively few passengers on modern airliners* develop such significant motion sickness that intervention is necessary.

For the most part, this is due to the more favourable meteorological circumstances in today's modern high-altitude flight levels. Even though one must ascend and descend "through the weather," particularly turbulent sectors can be avoided due to meteorological observation and advisories.

The cause of motion sickness symptoms lies in the discrepancy between optical, vestibular, and proprioceptive stimuli.

In particular, the exposure to non-controllable or unanticipated motion, especially when one is not prepared with proper head position, can result in a sudden appearance of symptoms.

Factors which initiate motion sickness from the perspective of the individual:

- Genetic disposition
- Intact vestibular system
- Poor training in the sense of a lack of experience with movement stimuli
- Influence of drugs (also nicotine and alcohol)

The following stimuli cause **particularly negative results**:

- Strong acceleration and deceleration components
- Rapid, unexpected position changes, especially vertical accelerations
- Movement around the lateral axis, especially forward
- Rapid or protracted movements around the longitudinal axis
- Noise
- Heat
- Olfactory stimuli

Common symptoms

- Apathy
- Sweating
- Hypersensitivity to smells and noise
- Heat intolerance
- Pallor
- Changes in salivation
- Nausea
- Vomiting

Recommendations and interventions for motion sickness during flight

- Sustain upright position especially during turbulence with significant vertical components
- Upright head position, optimally at a 30° forward inclination
- When supine, the head should be elevated
- Avoid significant head-down positions with the face down
- Avoid alcohol and nicotine (nicotine patches if needed)
- Avoid reading or working on a laptop computer
- Avoid head movements during turbulence
- Visual focus on a fixation point outside the aircraft; alternatively, closing eyes
- With *nausea and vomiting, metoclopramide (MCP)*, e.g. 10 mg administered intravenously

Recommendations and medication prophylaxis

- Sensitive individuals should consult with their physicians prior to flight and obtain medications
- Reserve a *seat in the middle of the aircraft*!
- Excluding contraindications for using *scopolamine* – e.g. in patch form for older children and adults (scopolamine TTS)
- Apply the patch *about 6 hours prior to flight* or the night before departure.

Alternatively, preparations with the ingredient *dimenhydrinate* can be considered and used like scopolamine as a therapeutic in the event that rapid treatment is needed, e.g. Vomacur tablets or Vomex A 150 suppositories.

4   Fear of flying

Fear of flying is a common phenomenon for adults. Frightening memories or a previous traumatic experience seem to play a great role in primary fear of flying. While children are accustomed to trust others – adults – it is difficult for adults to do so, especially when they are used to being in control of themselves or others. In the airplane, they feel at the mercy of the technical aspects of flight and somewhat of the crew. In three dimensions, they feel subjected to the forces of gravity, the engines, the weather, the aerodynamic acceleration processes, the spoiler (air brakes) and, after landing, to the reverse thrust.

Estimates and questionnaires indicate that *at least 30% of all airline passengers suffer from fear of flying*, some permanently, many under specific flight circumstances, and many merely during particular life stages, or depending on day-to-day condition. There is a number of people, as indicated above, whose fear is so great *before* flight that they will not attempt to determine whether they will experience fear *during* flight.

Seminars to overcome fear of flying

For many decades, successful seminars have been offered in Germany and around the world to overcome fear of flying. During such weekend programmes, the participants receive, among other information, details on the construction and aerodynamics of aircraft and information regarding technical maintenance and servicing. Additionally, the particular criteria for crew selection and the high level of education and training components for passenger care are described.

The seminar participants learn how thoroughly modern commercial aviation is handled technically and organizationally so that there is little to worry about with regard to the abovementioned concerns. Finally a short round-trip flight is taken together.

In this manner, individuals with primary fear of flying can enjoy flight and, by participating in these seminars, learn to trust the technical and operational aspects in order to control their unpleasant feelings.

Those who are not affected as strongly, or those who may have no choice but to "get over it" due to their occupations, account for a large figure of unreported cases among airline passengers who, under certain circumstances and possibly during a single flight, would actually need medical intervention.

Symptoms of fear of flying on board

- Restlessness and aggressiveness (so-called "unruliness": insubordinate, obstinate behavior), often combined with high alcohol consumption
- Hyperventilation
- Panic attack
- Psychovegetative dysregulation (sweating, tachycardia, hypertension)
- Combination of these symptoms

In general, all medical evaluations on board should determine whether a case of fear of flying exists, as the investigation of this determination alone may be the most important part of solving the problem.

Intervention for hyperventilation

It is important to normalize the respiratory frequency and depth of breathing by:

- Calm verbal intervention
- Leading the breathing in a measured pace as well as conscious diaphragmatic breathing
- Medical sedation with a benzodiazepine (midazolam 1–5 mg or diazepam 2.5–10 mg administered intravenously)

See also Chapter III.6.3, Hyperventilation.

Panic attack

A panic attack or mixed psychosomatic symptoms are usually controlled reasonably well, e.g. hyperventilation through an empathetic approach with a calm and open *conversation* – possibly also using *medical sedation*.

The on-board medical kit, depending on the airline, usually contains *benzo-diazepines and/or neuroleptics* as intravenous medications. Dosage depends on the severity of the symptoms and whether the patient has experience with the medications. A general guideline is:

- ½ to 1 ampoule (5–10 mg) diazepam
- In a psychotic presentation with altered perception and hallucinations, in combination with 1–2 ampoules (5–10 mg) haloperidol, intramuscular or intravenous
- If necessary, repeat dosage within a short period of time (15–30 minutes)

In the event that the neuroleptic haloperidol produces extrapyramidal reactions, such as torticollis, intramuscular or slow intravenous injection of ½ to 1 ampoule (2.5–5 mg) Akineton® is the treatment of choice.

Alcohol intoxication

A more difficult situation exists when there is heavy alcohol ingestion with uninhibition and aggressiveness. If necessary, and with the agreement of the crew and other passengers, *coordinated physical restraint* may be applied.

In some cases, airline captains have had to exercise their *power of authority* on board. With respect to the patient, the physician on board should also act as an advocate for the other passengers and crew. In order to keep other passengers, perturbed by an agitated and aggressive fellow traveller, out of harm's way, a courageous "doctoral intervention" may be reasonable and necessary.

5   Cardiovascular emergencies on board

In contrast to popular opinion, serious cardiovascular events are rather uncommon on board commercial aircraft. Approximately 75 million passengers are transported annually by Lufthansa German Airlines AG, and in the year 2012 physician assistance was requested a total of approximately 2,000 times. This translates into an illness rate of 0.002% of passengers with 40% cardiovascular and neurological symptoms. Of these, only 6% (n = 70 corresponding to 0.00013% of passengers) suffered from a potentially life-threatening cardiovascular condition.

Medical assistance from either a physician or healthcare professional was available in more than 80% of cases. Considering life expectancy, one can extrapolate that of 75 million passengers annually on board Lufthansa aircraft, there should theoretically be 350 on-board deaths every year if the figure were to correspond to the death rate of a medium-sized German town. In reality, there are approximately 10 on-board deaths per year.

For cardiopulmonary resuscitation *on board, see Chapter IV.*

5.1   Circulatory collapse and unconsciousness

The most common cardiovascular incident on board is simple circulatory collapse. Of the 1,126 total medical incidents on Lufthansa flights in 2004, 760 were traceable to this type of situation.

A variety of causes can lead to the so-called vasovagal syncope. In contrast to ground-based emergency care, there is rarely any evidence of a cardiovascular condition as the source of this type of loss of consciousness in the flight environment.

> More often, the majority of syncopal episodes are manifestations of a protracted travel-related illness, acute diarrhoea, or fear of flying.

Negatively perceived stimuli, such as passive and three-dimensional motion, mismatch of optical and vestibular input, mild hypoxia, and physical fatigue from lengthy travel can lead to vegetative overload and regulatory compromise in sensitive individuals. Stimulation of the nausea centre in the medullary postrema region leads to elevated vagal tone. Cognitively, feelings of insecurity, negative expectations, or outright fear of flying can be significantly strengthened by cortical influences. Skin pallor, profuse sweating, nausea or vomiting signify cutaneous or gastrointestinal symptoms.

Neurological dysregulation of vascular resistance and capacity result in a reduction in preload on the one hand and a loss of arterial resistance on the other. Additionally, in some individuals, a reflex bradycardia can be produced. All these named mechanisms lead to a restriction of cerebral circulation. Below a critical threshold of cerebral perfusion, a loss of autoregulation rapidly results in decreased mentation or a full loss of consciousness.

Intervention in circulatory collapse

Initial treatment necessitates lying down flat and, most importantly, elevating the legs above the head and thorax. In a suitable business class seat, treatment may be performed in the patient's seat. In economy class, the lack of space necessitates a supine position on a blanket on the floor, in the galley or the emergency exit area. It is important to select the treatment area carefully in the event that the condition worsens and escalates to resuscitation, so that neither passengers, equipment nor other assistants are in the way.

Basic measures for the unconscious patient
- Immediate extrication from the seat to the nearest place where resuscitation can take place (galley, aisle, or area by the exit doors)
- Adequate room at the head of the patient (intubation) and to the side of the chest (proper heart massage)
- Basic check for: responsiveness, breathing, pulse

- Supine position for cardiac insufficiency (caveat: acute cardiac insufficiency, brain haemorrhage), lateral decubitus position for decreased protective reflexes if CPR not required

Intervention for vasovagal syncope

For simple vasovagal syncope, the *aforementioned positions* result in an autotransfusion of about 300–500 ml blood from the venous system in the legs which is usually adequate to reestablish consciousness.

Circulatory insufficiency is the cause of **persistent unconsciousness,** and after verification (blood pressure measurement, pulse rate and quality), intravenous access with a rapid infusion of 500 ml crystalloid solution (Jonosteril® in the Doctor's Kit) as soon as possible is of primary importance.

Prior to volume infusion, one should *rule out overt or compensated cardiac insufficiency* as the primary cause.

Supplemental *oxygen* (4 l/min) is indicated.

Sympathomimetics should only be given after exhausting all of these possibilities (on board, Suprarenin® (epinephrine) is available, carefully (diluted) titrated intravenously under ECG monitoring: Be prepared to provide CPR).

Clarification of sudden loss of consciousness

In emergency medical aid, the prompt treatment of life-threatening disorders is just as important as the rapid differential diagnosis of the underlying problem.

> The initial diagnosis is and remains the working hypothesis which the results of examination and effects of treatment verify. In this respect, every emergency situation is a highly dynamic intellectual process.

Differential diagnosis of sudden loss of consciousness

- Vasovagal syncope, see above
- Cardiac arrest
- Symptomatic cardiac dysrhythmias
- Hypoglycaemic shock – see Chapter III.7.2
- Cerebrovascular accident (ischaemia, haemorrhage) – see Chapter III.7.1
- Seizure – see Chapter III.7.3
- Intoxication (drugs, medications, poisoning)

A reliable evaluation of pulse, blood pressure, and respiration is just as important as an obligatory blood glucose determination and assessment of the neurological status.

Neglecting these fundamentals by attributing "harmless syncope" to a case of prolonged hypoglycaemia can result in an apallic syndrome as deleterious as cardiac arrest.

For cardiopulmonary resuscitation *on board, see Chapter IV.*

5.2 Tachycardia

In order to diagnose tachyarrhythmias, emergency medicine physicians ask two critical questions:

1. Is the tachycardia symptomatic?
2. What time frame and operational possibilities are available to make a diagnosis and specify treatment?

In addition, it must be determined if the cardiac arrhythmia is a reflection of an underlying medical disorder or if it is secondary to a treatable illness. Tachycardia often appears as the compensatory tachycardia arising from other conditions:

- Reflex tachycardia in painful conditions or internal medical conditions (such as pulmonary embolus or cardiac decompensation during acute myocardial ischaemia)

Usually this is related to a morphological sinus tachycardia or a tachycardia absoluta. Here the treatment is focused on the underlying medical condition.

Immediate treatment is necessary for patients with:

- Rapid or weak pulse
- Signs of cardiovascular or neurological decompensation
- Dyspnoea at rest, pulmonary oedema, disturbance of consciousness, or angina pectoris

First aid for life-threatening tachycardia includes

- Supplemental oxygen
- Preparation for CPR
- Position that assists circulation

If circulation is adequate and consciousness is maintained, a *semi-seated position* with elevated thorax (e.g. support by cushions or further assistants) and legs lowered is preferred. In general, this is the position of choice for dyspnoeic patients and in many cases urgently demanded by the patient. Reducing the respiratory effort and workload, this position offers a mild decrease in cardiac preload and acutely reduces central congestion.

In *volume-depleted conditions* and during cardiogenic shock, *a supine position* can be advantageous for cardiac output.

Hopefully, characteristic clinical symptoms on board assist in making the correct determinations.

Proper places for such positioning:

- *Business class seat* in direct proximity to the galley (remain prepared for resuscitation!)
- *Empty seat row near an emergency exit*
- A large and clear area in the *galley,* supported by pillows and cushions

As much as possible, the patient should not walk there but should be carried by two assistants in a proper manner.

Other immediate measures

- Venous access
- AED application (ECG diagnostics)

In this manner, the prerequisites for a more precise analysis of cardiac dysrhythmia are afforded.

Analysis of tachycardia and appropriate treatment options

The first diagnostic step is the differentiation between regular tachycardia with a normal sequence of P wave and QRS complex or irregular tachycardia. The second step determines, if a wide-complex or narrow complex tachycardia is present (see Tab. 9).

In the event of irregular tachycardia, it is most likely due to atrial fibrillation. Rarely is acute intervention necessary. As long as there are no cardiopulmonary contraindications and the high heart rate is poorly tolerated, then symptomatic treatment with a *betablocker* (metoprolol [Beloc®] 5 mg titrated intravenously) to control the heart rate may be attempted. Cardioversion is left up to the subsequent medical facility to perform if necessary.

Tab. 9   The most common tachycardias in emergency situations and pragmatic approaches regarding patterns and morphology of the chambers

Regular tachycardias
Narrow complex tachycardia (QRS < 120 ms): Sinus tachycardia (p-waves) Reentry tachycardia (i.e. WPW syndrome, AV node reentry) Atrial flutter with regular block (3:1, 2:1)
Wide complex tachycardia (QRS > 120 ms): Ventricular tachycardia Supraventricular tachycardia with aberrant conduction Supraventricular tachycardia with bundle branch block
Irregular tachycardia
Usually atrial fibrillation with rapid ventricular response Occasionally pseudoarrhythmia absoluta with significant extrasystole activity

Only rarely is a pseudoarrhythmia absoluta encountered. This is usually due to advanced cardiopulmonary disease with chaotic supraventricular or ventricular rhythm arising from significant chronic myocardial damage.

Among regular tachycardias, *ventricular tachycardia* (VT) is particularly important. It appears as wide complex tachycardia, is general a *life-threatening condition*, and in most cases is due to acute myocardial ischaemia.

Rapid frequencies usually quickly deteriorate to *ventricular fibrillation* and require immediate termination through *electric cardioversion,* performed on board by means of unsynchronized defibrillation (see below).

Moderate frequencies are often haemodynamically stable and tolerated by patients. This provides a window of time to adequately prepare for *medical cardioversion* (positioning, oxygen supplementation, intravenous access) with an injection of 300 mg Cordarex® (available on board as amiodarone solution, 2 amp. at 150 mg). Alternatively, depending on the airline, lidocaine (xylocaine 1–1.5 mg/kg of body weight) is available for this specific antiarrhythmic therapy.

Treatment of last resort: On-board electrical defibrillation is available along with sedation with diazepam. As opiates are not available, one must do without prior analgesia in serious situtations (ketamine is not desirable for an elective termination of tachyarrhythmia due to sympathomimetic effects).

It should be noted that the AED will only discharge upon detection of a rhythm that requires defibrillation and has a frequency over 180 bpm; the device cannot be manually overridden below this frequency.

The other tachycardias are of a *significantly less harmful nature* (see Fig. 31) even though the patient subjectively perceives them as very disconcerting. With the limited equipment on board, it is not always possible to differentiate between VT and a wide complex supraventricular tachycardia with certainty. The latter can be an expression of a commonplace supraventricular tachycardia with a bundle branch block or aberrant conduction, in which case cardioversion would be unnecessary, unsuccessful, and contraindicated.

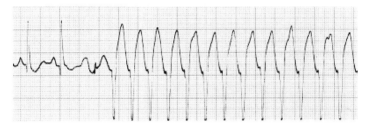

Fig. 31   Monomorphic ventricular tachycardia in a haemodynamically stable patient. Typical "hairpin" appearance of a wide complex tachycardia. Abnormal axis, AV dissociation (absence of regular sequence between P waves and QRS complex), appearance of so-called capture beats and fusion beats can delineate VT from supraventricular tachycardia with aberrant conduction or bundle branch block.

Reentry tachycardias most often occur in young people with healthy hearts who experience a sudden onset of a racing heartbeat. Occasionally a vagus manoeuvre (straining, coughing, drinking cold drinks) or a carotid sinus massage (after excluding atherosclerosis) can be helpful. Only rarely do reentry tachycardias lead to circulatory compromise, and usually they spontaneously terminate within minutes or in a few hours.

For cardiopulmonary resuscitation *on board, see Chapter IV.*

5.3   Hypertensive emergencies

Blood pressure crises are one of the most common acute situations in emergency medicine as well as on board. Situational influences such as fear, anger, fatigue, and physical causes such as motion sickness, pain, or acute internal conditions can lead to sudden dysregulation of blood pressure.

Primarily, it is necessary to distinguish between a hypertensive urgency (blood pressure over 220/120 mmHg without organic symptoms) and a *hypertensive emergency manifested by symptoms of organ damage*. These can appear as high pressure encephalopathy with stroke-like symptoms, acute left heart insufficiency, pulmonary oedema, or angina pectoris.

With asymptomatic hypertensive urgency, oral therapy with nitroglycerine (one puff oral spray or one oral capsule) or an oral calcium channel antagonist (Bayotensin® akut 1 ml solution for oral resorption [= 5 mg nitrendipine]) should be adequate.

Medical intervention in hypertensive crises

- Supplemental oxygen (4 l/min)
- Positioning with head and chest elevated
- Intravenous access
- Controlled blood pressure reduction (urapidil [Ebrantil®] 25 mg to 50 mg intravenously)

Initially Blood pressure should not be lowered by more than 15–20% of the initial value. If focal neurological signs are evident, blood pressure should be reduced to below 220 mmHg systolic, in this case not below 180/100 mmHg.

Blood pressure crises (like cardiac dysrhythmias) can be the initial symptom of another acute event:

- Cerebrovascular accident (accompanies about 50% of cases)
- Bleeding from a ruptured aneurysm, localization variable
- Myocardial infarction

Depending on the on-board availability, these should be clarified for each hypertension crisis. The question regarding the initial event cannot always be determined (similar to the "chicken and egg" question).

For all life-threatening events, *a diversion is* **recommended**.

5.4   ACS, angina pectoris and myocardial infarction

Due to the many possible complications, acute myocardial infarction is one of the most feared medical problems on board!

The reasons for this are the broad diagnostic uncertainties regarding classification of the nonspecific cardiac sympotomatology and the enormous potential for an *acute coronary syndrome* (ACS) to result in sudden death or rapid development of lethal cardiac insufficiency.

Acute coronary syndrome encompasses one of the following three constellations:
- Myocardial infarction with ST elevation on the ECG (STEMI)
- Myocardial infarction without ST elevation (NSTEMI)
- Unstable angina pectoris (UAP)

All three presentations have the same potential to result in *dangerous arrhythmia* which are primarily responsible for the high early fatality rate of ACS. In German pre-hospital care it is estimated, that about 30% of infarcted patients do not arrive at the hospital alive. 95–100% of these victims are affected by an infarct-induced cardiac dysrhythmia. Ventricular fibrillation (so-called primary VF) most commonly occurs within 24 hours (80% of the time) and most frequently within the first four hours. Therefore, immediate emergency medical treatment and intensive care monitoring are obligatory.

If a passenger complains of typical angina pectoris (AP) symptoms or the so-called AP equivalents (such as dyspnoea, nonspecific anxiety, or unexplained vegetative symptoms such as sweating or nausea), an acute emergency situation only can be considered excluded if it is a case of so-called stable AP. This is based on the premise that these symptoms are recognized by the patient and are the result of specific, identifiable triggers (exertion, excitement) and are entirely reversible (with rest or nitroglycerine within minutes).

> By contrast, every angina at rest – or first-time angina –, every continued AP lasting more than 20 minutes, every AP that is not improved with nitroglycerine, and every exacerbation of symptoms should be treated as acute coronary syndrome (ACS) and requires a heightened awareness regarding lethal cardiac dysrhythmias.

Physician's first response to acute coronary syndrome
- Immobilization, supine position with slight head and chest elevation (cardiac position, preferably in a business class seat near the galley)
- Oxygen by nasal cannula (4 l/min)
- Resuscitation equipment (complete emergency equipment with AED, Doctor's Kit)
- IV access with slow infusion (crystalloid)
- Continuous ECG monitoring with the AED
- Intubation equipment and emergency ampoule kit (particularly suprarenin, Cordarex®, and atropine) ready
- Aspisol 500 mg intravenously (possible contraindications: e.g. florid bleeding, asthma, anticoagulation therapy, pregnancy)
- Metoprolol 5–10 mg titrated intravenously (see below)
- Sedation (diazepam 5–10 mg intravenously)

For Analgesia – depending on blood pressure – a trial with *nitroglycerine*, e.g. two sublingual sprays or one sublingual capsule, can be undertaken. *Beta blockers* (metoprolol 5–10 mg titrated) provide analgesia and are protective against malignant cardiac dysrhythmias or an extension of the infarction. Contraindications for beta blockers like cardiac decompensation or conduction system disturbances must be considered. Opiates for analgesia are not available in the cabin pharmacy for understandable reasons.

> *ASC requires a* **diversion as soon as possible** *to the nearest airport with adequate medical facilities!*

Flying over Europe, one can count on a landing within 30 to 45 minutes. Long-distance flights over sparsely populated regions or oceans may span several hours before an airport with a qualified medical facility can be reached.

> **For cardiopulmonary resuscitation** *on board, see Chapter IV.*

5.5   Pulmonary embolism

The frequent appearance of thrombosis in relation to a flight, train ride, or road trip is generally due to the unavoidably long period of immobility. Pre-existing risk factors include thrombophilia, obesity, smoking, and a history of trauma, surgery, malignancy, pregnancy, hormone therapy and varicosis. In the case of flight, dehydration and mild hypoxia and subsequent release of nitric oxide (NO) from the endothelial tissues may facilitate a thrombosis.

In two of three randomized studies, the risk of thrombosis was elevated 2.3 to 4 times with flight; in a third study there was no statistically significant correlation. A consensus recommendation of the WHO suggested that flights less than three hours do not require any specific measures, and, without risk factors, advice pertaining to ingestion of adequate fluids (130 ml/h) plus engaging in repetitive activities such as isometric exercises, should be provided in the on-board information media, and should be adequate on longer flights. If there are any *risk factors,* Class I or II *compression stockings* should be worn, and *high risk individuals* should consider taking low molecular weight heparin two hours prior to flight.

If a thrombosis or consecutive pulmonary embolism develops, this is often silent and asymptomatic.

Only about 25% of lower extremity venous thromboses show any clinical symptoms. It is notable that 50% of all asymptomatic patients with proximal deep vein thrombosis (DVT) show evidence of pulmonary emboli on scintigraphy.

If a pulmonary embolus is symptomatic, the most common symptom (90%) is a *reflex tachycardia*. If a patient is found to have an unexplained "sinus tachycardia", an underlying pulmonary embolism may be present. The so-called "cor pulmonale" signs on the ECG (right axis rotation, S_IQ_{III} or $S_IS_{II}S_{III}$, right bundle branch block, ST changes in III, V1-V3, or P pulmonale) are diagnostically nondependable and not verifiable on board.

Symptomatology

Often the patient appears clinically *dyspnoeic* with normal auscultatory findings or minimal crackling noises. Possibly there are nonspecific complaints such as *chest pain* (70%), *fear or anxiety,* and cough. In about 15–30%, signs of circulatory compromise develop, with *sweating, syncope or frank shock*.

Medical intervention of pulmonary embolism with stable circulation

- Semi-supine position with elevated upper body
- Strict immobilization
- Intravenuous access with slow infusion (crystalloid)
- Supplemental oxygen (4 l/min)
- For mild dyspnoea, calm verbal intervention
- With severe dyspnoea, careful sedation with diazepam (Valium®) as long as adequate consciousness is maintained to support the increased respiratory effort

Targeted infusion of a narcotic in order to control breathing is logistically difficult on commercial aircraft.

Medical intervention upon suspicion of pulmonary embolism with circulatory compromise or evident shock

- As above
- Intubation equipment with emergency ampoule kit (particularly suprarenin, Cordarex® and atropine) ready
- Cardiopulmonary resuscitation measures depending on the situation (intubation, ventilation, heart massage)

> A severe pulmonary embolism has an unfavourable prognosis even on the ground; on board, the problem is compounded by the lower ambient air pressure and limited medical equipment.

The therapeutic benefit of intravenously administered Aspisol (ASS) is unproven. Thrombolytic therapy is usually not possible on board.

> *A severe pulmonary embolism is a clear indication for a medical diversion. Proper immobilization provides a greater range of discretion with mild or suspicious cases; however, most of the serious pulmonary emboli evolve over several stages, so that one must be prepared for significant worsening.*

5.6   Complications of pacemakers and ICDs

Patients with a pacemaker or ICD (implantable cardioverter defibrillator) should generally have their devices tested prior to the start of their trip and determine the servicing capabilities at their destination. Pacemaker interrogation before travelling is recommended, as is bringing along the required documentation (pacemaker card and, if necessary, a copy of the last pacemaker interrogation report).

Pacemaker complications on board are *rare* and in stable patients flights do not lead to an increased appearance of cardiac dysrhythmias that necessitate intervention. Due to the miniaturization and increasingly complex algorithms, hazardous pacemaker-induced tachycardia is hardly seen today.

> In the event of a hazardous pacemaker-induced tachycardia, the application of a permanent magnet on the implantation area is usually adequate to promptly stop the tachycardia.

ICD patients may fly, as long as their rhythm is stable and they do not anticipate any discharge (prophylactic implantation).

> In the event that repetitive shocks or anti-tachycardia stimulation occur during flight, the treatment availability on board, naturally, is very limited.

Depending on the situation, beta blockers are available for unstable ICD patients and, if necessary, other treatment options are amiodarone and sedatives such as *diazepam*.

6 Pulmonary problems

The only physiological difference between medical emergencies on board a commercial aircraft and a comparable situation on the ground is the *reduced ambient atmospheric pressure* and the associated *reduction in the partial pressure of alveolar oxygen*.

> **!** The reduced partial pressure of oxygen at flight altitudes can be completely and effectively compensated with supplemental medical oxygen. This simple measure should never be forgotten.

The low atmospheric pressure outside the aircraft at flight altitudes would result in loss of consciousness within 1–2 minutes and quickly lead to death. By pressurization, modern commercial aircraft maintain a comfortable and physiologically safe cabin pressure. According to regulations, the physical cabin pressure is maintained at a corresponding maximum altitude of 8,000 ft (2,438 m).

At this altitude, partial pressure of alveolar oxygen is reduced from 100 to 70 mmHg in healthy people, and the arterial oxygen saturation SaO_2 is reduced to 90%. This situation corresponds medically to mild hypoxia which is well tolerated without symptoms.

The cabin pressure, which corresponds to a mountain height of 2,500 m, may cause a healthy person to have mild symptoms, whereas a person with lung disease may experience significant dyspnoea. Those with chronic lung disease have adapted to a low arterial partial pressure of oxygen (see Fig. 32). Therefore it is important from an emergency medicine perspective to differentiate between acute and chronic respiratory insufficiency.

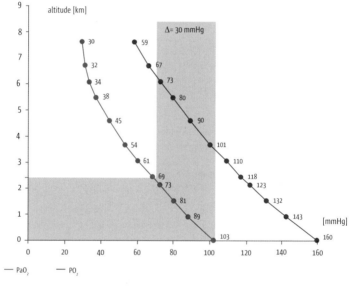

Fig. 32 Reduction of partial pressure of oxygen (left curve) and the total atmospheric pressure (right curve) with increasing altitude. A small altitude difference closer to the ground has a significantly greater effect than at higher altitudes. During ascent from sea level to cabin altitude (approx. 2,438 m) alveolar as well as arterial partial pressures are reduced by about 30%.

6.1 Bronchial asthma and asthma attacks

Asthma attacks on the ground as well as in the air must be taken very seriously. Even if the patient has a long history of mild asthma attacks, every new exacerbation has the potential to become a life-threatening situation.

Pathophysiologically speaking, bronchial asthma and exacerbations of chronic obstructive pulmonary disease (COPD) represent a pronounced *alveolar hypoventilation* due to a (partially) reversible bronchial obstruction. In contrast to diffusion disorders, alveolar hypoxia is often dramatically improved with oxygen.

This can be attained with simple supplemental oxygen. As long as the dyspnoeic patient tolerates it, oxygen is better administered by mask than by nasal prongs.

In combination with a reservoir bag, the inspiratory oxygen component can be increased from 21% up to 60%, thereby tripling the corresponding partial pressure.

An increase of the inspired oxygen concentration is *more effective at cabin altitude than on the ground*. Due to the exponential decrease in atmospheric pressure with increasing altitude, small altitude changes near the ground result in a significantly higher partial pressure loss than comparable altitude difference at e.g. 10,000 m. If the amount of loss of partial pressure between sea level and cabin altitude in the alveolar compartment is about 30 mmHg (in other words, about one third of the initial value), then by administration of oxygen the alveolar O_2 concentration can increase threefold, which is more than compensatory.

> Application of oxygen is the first action in emergency medicine. Its use on board a commercial airplane is particularly effective.

First aid for bronchial asthma
- Application of oxygen
- Calming by verbal intervention
- Instructions for slow and deep breathing
- Initiation of *pursed lip breathing* in order to increase intrinsic PEEP (positive end expiratory pressure)
- *Optimal positioning* to improve use of diaphragmatic and costal musculature

Whereas the chronic obstructive bronchitis is complicated by structural pulmonary changes with loss of alveolo-capillary gas exchange surfaces and bronchial collapse, the central and peripheral *ventilatory obstruction with bronchial asthma* is characterized by the following:

1. Muscular bronchospasm
2. Mucosal oedema with inflammatory infiltration
3. Dyscrinia with hypersecretion of thickened mucus

Medical intervention for asthma attacks

- **Prednisolone** 125–250 mg intravenously (preferably at the start of treatment). Due to their effect on the intracellular receptors followed by a transcription process, the steroids have a latency period of between 20 minutes and 4 hours before being effective. Then, they significantly accentuate the effects of beta-2 sympathomimetics on the receptor. Their dual action on muscular bronchospasm as well as on inflamed mucosa makes on-board treatment of the airway obstruction particularly effective.
- **Beta-2 sympathomimetics: Reproterol** (Bronchospasmin®) is available in the Doctor's Kit to treat acute airway obstruction.

Fenoterol (Berotec®), salbutamol (Sultanol®), or terbutaline (Bricanyl®), with predominantly bronchial effects, are the most potent bronchodilators available. For emergency treatment, one should exclusively use the *short-acting preparations*, as the effects of the long-acting derivatives (formoterol, salmeterol) begin to act after 20–30 minutes, and their delayed kinetics predispose to overdosage.

- **Adequate fluid replacement:** (2–3 l per 24 hrs) and *mucolytics* (from personal medical supply) to prevent mucostasis and dyscrinia (there are *no mucolytics* in the on-board pharmacy)
- **Respiratory therapy measures** (as is possible) for cough production and mucous mobilization

> Hypoxia and the simultaneous administration of multiple medications, which have cardiac effects (such as beta-2 agonists, theophylline) and a narrow therapeutic window, can lead to *serious cardiac dysrhythmias.* Often this is due to overdosing of emergency medications due to prior self medication use. Therefore it is obligatory to utilize the AED for cardiac rhythm monitoring.

6.1.1 Status asthmaticus

In refractory or life-threatening continued asthma attacks despite treatment with beta sympathomimetics, the treatment of last resort is:

- Initiation of a *Ketanest®/Dormicum® sedation* followed by
- Endotracheal intubation with manual bag ventilation

> *Severe dyspnoea or an inadequate response to treatment of airway obstruction within 10–20 minutes should be a generous indication for an unscheduled landing.*

6.2 Non-specific breathing problems

There is hardly any other symptom as ambiguous as the subjective perception of breathing difficulties. The challenge for the treating physician is the *history and differential diagnosis.*

With targeted and insistent *questioning* as well as careful observation of the ill person, it can be determined whether this is about true "air hunger", a feeling of anxiety in the chest, gastrointestinal distress, or an unconscious panic condition. Just as important are questions regarding preexisting conditions, associated somatic or vegetative symptoms, and the dynamics in which the complaints began.

> A sudden onset of shortness of breath can be an indicator of a serious internal medical condition such as a heart attack or pulmonary embolism.

With subtle worsening, one should consider a **psychogenic illness** or evolving infection such as pneumonia as being more likely.

> *Giving oxygen* in the majority of cases is reasonable and not harmful.

It improves hypoxia in patients with respiratory insufficiency. With organ infarction (myocardial infarction, stroke), it elevates and sustains the arterial oxygen partial pressure and thereby raises the effective pressure gradient for oxygen diffusion from the capillary bed into the hypoxic tissues.

Only in patients with **claustrophobic conditions** the application of an oxygen mask may aggravate the psychogenic symptoms. Holding the oxygen source in front of the face may be a good alternative in these cases.

Patients with **chronic respiratory insufficiency** should be monitored when given supplemental oxygen to avoid the (rare) development of asphyxia by overshooting CO_2 retention.

In addition to the specific treatment of the underlying medical conditions, *medical sedation* is often helpful to reduce the subjective perception of dyspnoea. This includes calming words, a calm and confident demeanor, as well as *empathetic communication* as tools of professional medical care.

6.3 Hyperventilation

Psychogenic factors are the predominant causes for a pathological increase in respiratory minute volume in the case of hyperventilation syndromes that require treatment. Particular triggers for exacerbation of phobias are the conditions on board a commercial airplane: the gathering of many people in a small space, the subjective unalterable motions in three-dimensional space, and, most recently, the fear of a terrorist attack. *Anxiety disorders with claustrophobic components, fear of flying or fear of heights* may play a particularly important role.

Indeliberate alveolar hyperventilation is difficult to control and rapidly leads to hypocapnia and respiratory alkalosis. The following shift in the free serum calcium due to increased binding to albumin results in a relative calcium deficiency, which leads to the so-called *"tetany symptoms"* (perioral and peripheral parasthesias, carpopedal spasms, etc.).

> Breathing into a plastic bag can rapidly resolve hypocapnia and tetany symptoms but does not provide any aetiological treatment for the psychogenic disturbance, particularly for the claustrophobic patient.

Intervention for hyperventilation

Normalization of respiratory rate and depth is improved with:

- Calm verbal intervention
- If necessary, leading breathing with a measured beat, deliberate diaphragmatic breathing, or
- Medical sedation with a benzodiazepine (such as midazolam 1–5 mg or diazepam 2.5–10 mg titrated intravenously)

> A tip from experienced flight attendants: One can take an oxygen bottle, slightly open the valve so that the air flow can be heard, and let the individual breath through a mask – the supplemental oxygen is inconsequential, but allows mild rebreathing to occur.

6.4   Pneumothorax

Spontaneous pneumothorax – pathological air in the pleural space with increasing encroachment onto respiration – is a rare event with an incidence of 18–28 per 100,000.

Clinically it presents with a sudden onset of chest pain, often accompanied by significant dyspnoea. However, it can also appear entirely without symptoms.

The cause in most cases are intrapulmonary emphysematous bubbles (so called "blebs"), which are predisposed to rupture and create an open air conduit ("air leak") between the bronchial system and the pleural space when they are located in the subpleural area.

The so-called tension pneumothorax presents a dramatic picture: Due to a valve effect (such as a unilateral pleural flap), air can enter through the bronchopleural fistula with each breath but cannot flow out. In this manner, the pneumothorax pumps itself up until the affected lung totally collapses and produces a mediastinal shift, which compromises the contralateral unaffected lung as well as the great mediastinal vessels.

Intervention in tension pneumothorax

This situation can turn life-threatening within minutes and requires immediate decompression by way of a *pleural puncture*. Because suction is not available, the disturbed mechanics of breathing must be supported by *positive pressure ventilation* (by way of endotracheal intubation and bag ventilation, alternatively by mask and sedation).

> *The first appearance of a pneumothorax on board is an* **absolute indication for landing** *as soon as possible.*

Physically, the reduction in cabin pressure during ascent leads to an expansion of the pathologic pleural air collection and can aggravate a previously existing pneumothorax. The volume of the gas trapped at sea level expands by a factor of about 1.4 at the cabin pressure present at high altitude flight levels.

Generally, only *rarely does a valve mechanism* develop in pneumothorax cases on the ground: In a British study, more than two days elapsed without complications in over 46% of patients with pneumothorax before they actually presented to a physician for treatment. Despite this potential for a serious mechanism, statistics show that in total only about 0.6 to 0.8% of all spontaneous pneumothorax episodes result in a lethal outcome.

7 Unconsciousness/seizures on board

Unexplained unconsciousness is a rare primary symptom on board, and its clarification is particularly difficult or even impossible, especially if there is no one to provide a history.

Basic evaluation of unconsciousness/seizure

- History! (accompanying relatives)
- Pulse, blood pressure, breathing
- Focused neurological examination
- Obligatory blood sugar determination

Clarification of sudden loss of consciousness

In emergency medicine, the immediate treatment of life-threatening disorders is just as important as the rapid differential diagnosis of the underlying cause.

> The initial diagnosis is the working hypothesis which the results of examination and effects of treatment verify. In this respect, every emergency situation is a highly dynamic intellectual process.

Differential diagnosis of sudden loss of consciousness
- Vasovagal syncope see Chapter III.5.1
- Cardiac/circulatory arrest or symptomatic cardiac arrhythmias see Chapter III.5.2
- Hypoglycaemic shock see Chapter III.7.2
- Cerebrovascular accident (ischaemia, haemorrhage) see Chapter III.7.1
- Seizure see Chapter III.7.3
- Intoxication (drugs, medications, poisoning)

On board, typical symptomatology will hopefully help to establish the correct interpretation.

7.1 Stroke/Transient ischaemic attack (TIA)

Symptoms

Clues to cerebral, usually ischaemic insults:
- Sudden or deteriorating appearance of speech impairments
- Arm or leg paresis or lateralizing symptoms

Hypertensive haemorrhages are less common.

Interventions for stroke/TIA
- Elevate head and chest, or stable lateral decubitus position
- Administer supplemental oxygen via nasal canula
- Establish peripheral venous access; if necessary, infuse electrolyte solution
- If blood pressure is severely elevated, IV titration of *urapidil* (Ebrantil®) utilizing the Doctor's Kit

Continuously monitor respirations for the rest of the flight and, if necessary, intubate to secure the airway.

Determine *blood glucose* in any event with the electronic blood glucose measuring device in the Doctor's Kit.

In most cases of cardiovascular compensated stroke or TIA continuing the flight to the final destination is desireable.

7.2 Hypoglycaemia

Hypoglycaemia as a possible cause of unconsciousness must always be considered!

Instructions for escorts of patients regarding the effects of blood sugar-lowering medications without adequate prior nutrition in known diabetics are helpful. Usually an attempt to give the patient glucose or a sugary drink or meal has already been undertaken.

In any event, the *actual blood glucose level* should be determined using either the electronic measuring unit in the *Doctor's Kit or the patient's own device*.

Intervention in critical hypoglycaemia/hypoglycaemic shock
- If unconscious, open and protect the airway
- Administer oxygen either via nasal canula or by mask
- Establish peripheral venous access; if necessary, infuse electrolyte solution
- administer 40% glucose slow intravenous push or into the running infusion

Ideally, the patient will awake and be responsive. Subsequently, attention should be paid to providing an adequate supply of glucose and, if necessary, further monitoring of blood glucose levels.

Usually the flight may continue to the destination, as long as the patient remains responsive and medical history can be obtained.

7.3 Seizures

Seizures in adults can be caused by subtherapeutic levels of medication in *known epileptics*, through *sleep deprivation* on long-distance flights, or, in rare cases, also by *alcohol withdrawal*.

Intervention during seizures
- Position the patient during the seizure in order to avoid further injury
- Protect from aspiration and tongue injury (Guedel tube fixated with tape)

If the seizure does not cease within a short period of time without taking measures:

- Midazolam 5–15 mg or diazepam 10–20 mg intravenously from the Doctor's Kit

The priority during the seizure is protection from secondary injury. To transfer the individual to the galley during an attack for treatment, such as to start an intravenous therapy, etc., is not possible within the confines of an airline cabin!

After giving an anticonvulsant, there should be *continuous monitoring of respiration* for the rest of the flight, stable lateral decubitus positioning, and, if necessary, supplemental oxygen by nasal cannula.

In any case, the actual *blood glucose level* should be determined with the electronic blood glucose device in the Doctor's Kit.

Usually the flight may continue to the destination if it is known that the patient has a seizure disorder. In the event that this is the first seizure, or with repeat episodes, a diversion should be considered following initial treatment.

8 Intoxication from alcohol, medications or drugs

Ingestion of *sedative medications* or overindulgence of alcohol can individually or in combination lead to loss of consciousness. Empty *pill bottles in the hand luggage* and/or the smell of alcohol (foetor alcoholicus ex ore) are often the only clues to the possible causes of the unconsciousness.

Intervention for intoxication from alcohol or medications
- Establish intravenous access and infuse an electrolyte solution from the Doctor's Kit
- Continuous monitoring of respiration for the duration of the flight
- Stable lateral decubitus positioning
- Oxygen via nasal cannula
- If patient is responsive, additional detoxification with oral fluids (fruit or herbal tea – no black tea or coffee!), 1–2 litres per hour to force diuresis

In any case, the actual *blood glucose level* should be determined with the electronic blood glucose device in the Doctor's Kit.

Usually it is possible to continue the flight to the destination!

Drug-induced emergency

Rarely a serious and life-threatening *drug intoxication* can occur. Usually these occur in drug couriers on flights from South or Central America to Europe. They have packed large amounts of illegal drugs inside their intestines preserved in packets. If such a packet breaks open, rapid resorption occurs with the typical signs of a drug overdose. This situation is absolutely life-threatening.

Treatment options are not available on board. One is limited to establishing intravenous access and infusing the available 4 x 500 ml electrolyte solutions to initiate diuresis. If possible, on should also provide oral fluids.

Of course, imminent respiratory failure should be treated with artificial respiration (intubation).

An immediate diversion is recommended. Only in a hospital setting life-saving treatment can be installed!

9 Food poisoning

Food poisoning is an overly dramatized occurrence in films rather than a frequent incident in real life.

Symptoms typically begin about six to ten hours after a contaminated meal – the incubation period is strongly dependent on the amount of the ingested food and the degree of bacterial contamination. After non-specific abdominal complaints, significant nausea develops leading to vomiting within a short period of time. Accompanying these symptoms are intestinal cramps with bloating, which is due to the gas expansion according to the Boyle-Mariotte law, and are thoroughly uncomfortable but not dangerous. If diarrhoea occurs, it develops hours later.

Treatment is entirely symptomatic. If needed, antiemetics (Vomacur®) and spasmolytics (Buscopan® supp.) can be given from the pharmacy. The patient should be positioned to comfort. It is important to provide adequate *supplemental fluids,* normally herbal tea, which is available from the galley. There is an additional soothing gastrointestinal effect from fennel tea. A rule of thumb is to provide about three cups (300 ml) of fluid per hour. Application of moist heat to the abdomen can also ameliorate colicky pain (hot water bottle wrapped in very warm, wet napkins, placed inside a dry towel).

As mentioned above, food poisoning is very uncommon. The catering services prepare the food under highest hygienic standards. Meals are carefully chilled or shock-frozen, and the refrigerator is locked until it is brought onto the airplane. Food that is particularly sensitive to bacterial contamination, such as mayonnaise or clams, are not served on board. In addition, a sample of each order is frozen and retained for at least ten days after preparation. In the event that there is an episode of food poisoning on board, it can be determined if the meal was the cause.

Generally, only individual cases occur. In the rare event of a mass infection, the situation is different. The limited facilities, such as the number and availability of restrooms on board, the unanticipated consumption of fresh water, running out of drinks, etc., can lead to an unscheduled landing in such a highly unlikely situation.

Food poisoning is an extremely rare occurrence. Treatment is symptomatic. A diversion – with the exception of a mass infection – does not usually need to be considered!

10 Choking from foreign body aspiration on board (adults)

Accidental *aspiration* of a bolus or foreign body results in a sudden mechanical obstruction of the trachea. The patient can only cough the bolus out if it has been aspirated during the end of an inspiratory phase.

> As soon as it is evident that the patient cannot cough or breathe, rapid and focused treatment is necessary as there are only 2–3 minutes available!

Intervention for bolus aspiration – Adults

In a calm manner and with few words, the problem should be explained to the patient while the following *measures* are undertaken:

- Attempt using multiple sharp strikes between the patient's shoulder blades
- Preparation for intubation!
- Application of the Heimlich manoeuvre in the standing or supine patient: multiple abdominal thrusts with both hands on the epigastrium – five times – then inspection of the mouth and throat (success is rare!)

- If unsuccessful, attempt to remove the foreign body with Magill forceps or by suctioning
- If this, too, is unsuccessful: Endotracheal intubation, attempt to extract bolus by suctioning
- Treatment of last resort: With the endotracheal tube, attempt to push the bolus beyond the bifurcation of the trachea into (usually the right) bronchus, then retract the tube into the mainstem bronchus and block – only for experienced emergency medical responders!
- In the case of an irreversible laryngeal obstruction by a bolus, which cannot be removed, or in the case of (e.g. allergic) oedema, a tracheal puncture with a wide-lumen IV catheter or even a tracheal incision should be considered

Clearly, all aspiration conditions that cannot be controlled and result in a continued limitation of breathing are reason for a diversion!

11 Colics

11.1 Biliary colic

In the USA, about 20% of women and 8% of men over the age of 40 have gall stones. Depending on nutritional habits, Europeans and Asians, especially Japanese, are substantially less afflicted with cholelithiasis than US Americans.

Acute symptoms often appear due to:

- Cholecystitis
- Gall duct colic specifically; i.e. the incarceration of a concretion in the cystic duct or in the common bile duct

Particularly **affected** are overweight women (about twice as often as men) of western provenance and of middle age. Often after a (fatty) meal, usually in the evening or at night (time zone changes during flight!) or during the day, a pressure feeling occurs in the upper abdomen with loss of appetite and well-being. Often previous episodes are revealed when questioned about symptoms.

Symptoms

Particularly with a *stone obstruction, cramping right upper abdominal pain* can rapidly develop with radiation along the right costal margins into the interscapular region, or the right scapular or shoulder area, accompanied by nausea and vomiting.

If the stone occludes the common bile duct, icterus with pruritus can develop within a few hours, which verifies the diagnosis. The affected person suffers from significant right upper abdominal pain, is often pale, sweating, and is subfebrile or febrile.

The examination reveals tenderness in the right upper quadrant with localized guarding.

Differential diagnosis in adults

Duodenal ulcer: typically no radiation of pain, no elevated temperature, usually thin males rather than overweight females, usually improved after eating, rarely rapid escalation of symptoms resulting in colic and vomiting; significant symptom acceleration and board-like abdomen are signs of perforation

Posterior wall infarct: sagittal radiation between the shoulder blades, no temperature elevation, often a fear of death, possibly more pronounced circulatory symptoms, collapse, dyspnoea, and cardiac dysrhythmias

Right-sided renal colic: flank pain, radiation of pain to the lower abdomen, usually affecting males, no elevation of temperature, no apathy but rather an urge to move

Pancreatitis: point of maximal pain usually in the mid-abdomen with radiation to the back, squeezing or knife-like pain, soft abdomen, flaccid abdominal wall, and significant fever if protracted

Intervention for gall bladder colic
- No food intake except oral fluid intake in small sips
- If necessary, IV infusion
- Analgesia initially with 1 amp. novaminsulfon intravenously
- Spasmolysis with 1 amp. Bucospan® intravenously

Spasms often respond quickly to *nitrolingual* (1–2 capsules or 1–2 sublingual application, repeat if necessary).

11.2   Renal and urinary colic

Primarily affected are adults between the ages of 20 and 60 years – men approx. 50% more often than women. About 5% of all adults experience one or more kidney stone episodes. The recurrence rate within 10 years is about 50%. Insufficient fluid intake predisposes to renal stone colics.

Often the symptoms described in an exact anamnesis already allow a clear diagnosis. Because of the high recurrence rate, it is important to ask about prior episodes!

Symptoms

Colicky pain is usually quite *severe*, develops rapidly, and manifests itself within 20–60 minutes as a *severe, sharp, recurring, or continual pain, which* patients are literally convulsing with. In contrast to pain from other causes, the patient usually is not apathetic, but has an urge to move which can be utilized therapeutically.

Pain localization is strongly unilateral right or left and, *depending on the position of the stone,* is either higher or lower in the Head's zones of the kidney and ureters, i.e. dorsally paravertebral at the level of the caudal ribs or more along the flank to the lower abdomen. Even if the pain is perceived in the region of the flank, one should ask about further radiation of pain! With prevesicular ureteral stones on the right, one should consider the *differential diagnosis of appendicitis, in which case* pain is less severe, usually initially in the epigastrium, and not originating in the region of the flank.

Intervention for renal stones in the region of the kidney and ureters

Even on board a commercial aircraft, a definitive diagnosis can be made, leading to focused and pragmatic treatment:

- Generous *hydration* by the litre; even alcoholic drinks in the form of beer are allowed here!
- Caveat: Caffeine-containing drinks such as coffee, tea, or enriched energy drinks in combination with mild hypoxia can lead to acute urinary retention!
- *Spasmolysis* with 1 amp Bucospan® IV, repeat if needed
- *Analgesia* wit Novaminsulfon 5 ml or Tramal® 2 ml intravenously
- *Movement*, if possible by hopping in place, or up and down stairs. It should be noted that Lufthansa's long-range aircraft, B747, some A 330/340 and the A380, have at least one set of stairs.

This regimen does not always result in a spontaneous resolution, but nonetheless is successful in about 70% of cases. The aforementioned treatment provides pain reduction so that the patient has some relief and that the flight can continue without a diversion. Of course, the patient must be advised to estimate his *urinary volume* so that it can be matched to the fluid intake to recognize a developing acute *urinary retention*.

Only in the case of severe pain, urinary retention (!) or development of fever it is necessary to consider a diversion, depending on the remaining flight distance and available medical facilities at the diversion airport!

12 Injuries and burns

12.1 Scalding and burns

Injuries certainly occur on board and they may well be due to carelessness of the passenger and are sometimes a direct result of blatant disregard of recommendations or regulations. Burns, on the other hand, are quite uncommon. The famous "coffee situation" with hot liquid spilling onto the passenger during on-board service rarely occurs.

However, burns are certainly an issue for the *flight attendants*. During meal preparation, due to the narrow galleys, the hot ovens, and hurried, improper or careless handling of the hot trays, burns can occur which usually affect the hand and forearm.

First and foremost, *cooling of the burn* is indicated, e.g. with cold water.

It is not a good idea to take a small piece of dry ice, used in the galley for food and beverage chilling, to wrap it in a towel and apply it to the area. The towel will stick to the wound, and the severe cold of the dry ice will lead to frostbite!

As usual, the *wound* should be covered with sterile material, blisters should not be opened, and the affected *extremity should be kept at rest*. Moreover it should be kept elevated in order to promote blood and lymph drainage subsequently reducing oedema and the ensuing pain from swelling. The appropriate bandages and other materials can be found in the *First Aid Kit.*

12.2 Injuries

In contrast, injuries are much more common among passengers than among flight attendants. They range from sprains when going from the aisle to the cabin, to scalp lacerations from luggage falling from overloaded overhead bins, to fractures of the extremities and ribs.

> Despite the flight attendants' suggestion, the overhead bins are stuffed full. A minor amount of turbulence is enough to shake the airliner and warp it slightly, which can open the latches of the bins. One can imagine what happens when a 10 kg hard case cosmetic bag drops onto a passenger's head from a height of 60 cm!

> *During night flights,* the cabin is darkened to give the passengers an opportunity to sleep, watch a movie, or even to work. The relative darkness creates a hazard for *tripping* in the aisle. This is made worse by the other passengers who put purses or camera bags, or even newspapers or magazines, in the aisle. If one is a bit groggy from awakening from sleep, one can be somewhat disoriented and unsteady on the feet. This situation is exacerbated in the aircraft types Airbus A 340–600 in that the restrooms are no longer spread out over several places in the cabin but are located in concentrated areas. One such location is on the lower deck and requires the use of stairs, with a step height and depth unlike that usually found in buildings.

Sprains

A sprain can be treated with on-board measures: cooling, rest, immobilization, and if needed, pain medication.

Fractures

The most common cause is severe turbulence, which is not always predictable, as in the case of so-called *clear air turbulence* (CAT). These meteorological events can result in dropping commercial aircraft the size of a B747 a few hundred metres within seconds. All loose objects as well as unsecured passengers will then be tossed around the cabin, thrown against the ceiling and pressed against the floor.

Fractures of the extremities are usually the result. Even in less severe forms, but nonetheless sufficient to result in such injuries, numerous such events occur annually worldwide, some of which lead to an unscheduled landing.

There are *semi-elastic splints* made out of plastic which can be shaped into stable forms and are useful for *immobilization*. These can be held in place with an elastic wrap.

Open fractures must, of course, be handled to remain sterile. Repositioning of dislocated fractures should probably not be performed as this is usually unsuccessful due to the severe pain it can cause, thereby potentially worsening any symptoms of shock.

Transport to an appropriate location and *positioning* are the most important challenges. A supine position, especially with a lower extremity fracture, is necessary. A first or business class seat should therefore be utilized as they afford more possibilities for positioning. This will also leave more room for a physician to work. Transporting a passenger through the narrow aisles of the airplane is not an easy task – in addition to the physical demand on the physician and assistant, the ability to perform the *Rautek grip* (special rescue manoeuvre) is a requirement in order to avoid secondary injury or create a shock situation.

For intervention in the event of delayed *shock* and to provide efficient *pain management* including *sedation,* it is necessary to establish venous access in all cases.

In certain cases of immobility, movement inside the aircraft may not be possible due to the extent of the injury, such as a spiral fracture of the femur. Here it is recommended that the patient be pulled onto a *blanket spread on the cabin floor* and then dragged to the nearest, accordingly prepared galley (first securing all trolleys and equipment, etc.) and positioned there. The injured person will lie perpendicular to the direction of flight against the fore wall padded with blankets and pillows to prevent any slipping. This will provide the most protection during landing and braking.

This is the limit of the therapeutic possibilities in aircraft. A diversion for medical reasons can be taken into consideration for very unusual cases. Serious soft tissue injuries are conceivably associated with uncontrollable venous or arterial blood loss.

13 Problems and emergencies with children

Emergencies with healthy children are rarely seen on board of commercial aircrafts. In general, one must make sure that the children are occupied, drink sufficiently, and are dressed warm enough (see Chapter I.1).

Being aware of the special characteristics of aviation medicine, one should first consider the problems of the upper airway, especially concerning ear pain. Children, especially infants, are significantly more sensitive in this aspect than adults.

13.1 Ear, nose, and throat infections in children

When informed about an upper airway infection, one should first prescribe the previously neglected first aid measures. Now, warm drinks are better than cold ones.

When ear pain presents, one should immediately instill nasal drops into both nostrils, which, depending on the length of the flight, may need to be generously repeated. It may also be necessary to provide analgesia; use paracetamol for young children and aspirin with older children. This may also require multiple repeat doses. Treatment for acute *sinusitis* is similar.

Intervention for otalgia and acute sinusitis

Infants:
- nasal drops, e.g. Otriven® 0.05% each dropper
- Paracetamol supp. 125 mg

Young children:
- nasal drops, e.g. Otriven® 0.05% each dropper
- Paracetamol supp. 250 mg

School-age children:
- nasal drops, e.g. Otriven® 0.05% each dropper
- Paracetamol supp. 250–500 mg
- ASS 250–500 mg (*caveat*: allergy)

It is important to establish pressure equalization before the aircraft begins descent.

During the entire descent, it is important that the child regularly swallows, chews gum, and yawns actively in order to establish pressure equalization. Once the middle ear is under-pressurized, it is nearly impossible to treat with on-board measures.

13.2 Fever and febrile seizures in children

In the event of fever, the same rules apply as on the ground:
- First calm the child and its mother. Fever is a necessary physiological response of the body.
- Only when the fever rises *above 39.5–40° C*, or with a history of febrile seizures, should one generously administer *paracetamol* in the above-mentioned doses, up to four times per day.

In the event of a *febrile seizure*, rectal or intravenous *diazepam* is the treatment of choice.

Intervention for febrile seizure

Infants:
- Diazepam Desitin® rectal 5–10 mg
- Valium® 2–5 mg IV

Young children:
- Diazepam Desitin® rectal 10–20 mg
- Valium® 5–10 mg IV

13.3 Abdominal pain in children

Particular diagnostic difficulties can arise regarding the evaluation of *abdominal pain* in infants and younger children. It is, again, important to establish and maintain a calm atmosphere.

If the complaints are generally *periumbilical*, the tongue is moist, and the abdominal wall is soft without any resistance, then one can give medications to provide relief and wait.

One should not expect to be able to evaluate bowel sounds by auscultation in a noisy flight environment.

Treatment initially consists of *local warmth* and *withholding of food and, if necessary, of fluids*. Should bloating be determined – an entirely expected phenomenon – then 10–20 drops of *metoclopramide* may be given orally.

Analgesics and spasmolytics only after determination of diagnosis!

The *administration of analgesics* and, if necessary, of spasmolytics, should only be undertaken if one is sure enough of the diagnosis and the complaint of pain seems to necessitate it.

Infants:

- Paracetamol supp. 125 mg
- Buscopan® ½ supp. or
- Buscopan® s.c. or slow intravenous push, 0.3 mg–0.6 mg/kg (maximum daily dose: 1.5 mg/kg)

Young children:

- Paracetamol supp. 250 mg
- Buscopan® ½ to 1 supp. or
- Buscopan® s.c. or slow intravenous push, 0.3 mg–0.6 mg/kg (maximum daily dose: up to 1.5 mg/kg)

School-age children:

- Paracetamol supp. 250–500 mg
- If necessary, Tramal® s.c. or slow intravenous push (1–2 mg/kg for children over one year of age)
- Buscopan® 1 supp. or
- Buscopan® s.c. or slow intravenous push, 0.3 mg–0.6 mg/kg (maximum daily dose: up to 1.5 mg/kg)

Acute abdomen in children

Regarding additional symptoms such as repetitive *vomiting, unconsciousness,* or accelerating signs such as abdominal resistance to palpation, generalized pressure, *peritoneal signs, and a rigid abdomen,* a serious illness must be presumed.

The diagnosis of an acute abdomen must be discussed with the cockpit crew and, if necessary, an unscheduled landing planned, taking into account whether the diversion destination can be expected to have adequate treatment facilities.

13.4 Choking fits (children)

Acute respiratory distress in young children is usually caused by one of the following:
- Foreign body aspiration in 20%
- Bronchial asthma in 20%
- Pseudocroup in 40%

Particularly in young children, aspiration of a food bolus or foreign body, such as a small toy, can result in an airway obstruction.

13.4.1 Foreign body aspiration

A sudden mechanical obstruction of the trachea in the deeper bronchial tree occurs. The little patient immediately develops a severe cough and respiratory distress.

Intervention for aspiration (child)

Both the child and the parent should be told in a very calm manner what the problem is while the following measures are being undertaken:
- *Prepare for intubation* if respiratory distress and cyanosis are present
- *Inspect the oral cavity* – if possible, remove the foreign body
- *Infant:* several (moderate) taps between the shoulder blades with the child in a head-down position with its abdomen on the thigh of the responder (no Heimlich procedure!)
- *Young and school-age child:* initial attempt with several soft to medium-heavy blows between the shoulder blades
- *Young child/toddler:* position the child on its back on a firm surface and give 5–10 upper abdominal thrusts

- *School-age child*: application of the *Heimlich manoeuvre* in the standing or supine position; multiple thrusts on the epigastrium
- Repeat *inspection of the oral cavity*, to assess whether mechanical intervention was successful
- If unsuccessful, attempt *mask breathing* (100% O$_2$)
- If not possible, attempt foreign body removal with *Magill forceps*
- If unsuccessful, intubate and attempt to suction out the bolus *or*
- Treatment of last resort: attempt to push the bolus distally with the endotracheal tube into (usually the right mainstem) bronchus, then retract the tube into the trachea. Caveat: only for trained emergency responders!
- In the event of an *irreversible obstruction of the laryngeal region by a bolus* which cannot be removed or due to (e.g. allergic) *oedema*, a *tracheal puncture with a wide-lumen IV catheter* or even a *tracheal incision* should be considered

In children, a complete upper airway obstruction is uncommon, but deep breathing with cough and otherwise adequate respiratory function can be expected, and positioning, supplemental oxygen and sedation should be considered.

Further treatment

- For stable respirations without cough, no further measures are needed
- If applicable, extubate
- If necessary, supplemental oxygen
- If necessary, theophylline 5-6 mg/kg slow IV push
- If necessary, Rectodelt® (prednisolone) 100 mg rectal
- If necessary, sedation with ¼–½ Diazepam Desitin® rectal tube

It is obvious that all aspiration situations that are not controlled and result in continued respiratory distress must lead to a diversion!

13.4.2 Pseudocroup – Subglottal laryngotracheitis

Small children between the age of 6 months and 4 years can be afflicted with a (usually viral) *subglottal laryngotracheitis* causing a stenosis due to mucosal swelling in the small diameter airway. Pseudocroup causes one third of *respiratory distress* in the above-mentioned age groups.

Pseudocroup appears primarily in the cold season and develops gradually. The children initially have a preceding *inspiratory stridor* and are often unencumbered; their temperature is usually between *subfebrile to febrile*.

Intervention for Pseudocroup

- Calming of the child and especially the parents
- Do not separate from the main attachment person
- Sitting position is better than lying down
- Humidify the air through cool, moist towels
- Sufficient fluid intake: cold drinks (decongestant)
- Administration of 1 supp. Rectodelt® (prednisolone) 100 mg by the attachment person
- Possibly up to 125 mg Solu-Decortin (4 mg/kg) IV
- Possibly provide supplemental oxygen
- Avoid sedation

If stabilization does not occur, early contact with the cockpit crew should be established in order to recommend a diversion. This particularly applies if there is a suspicion of epiglottitis (stenosing supraglottal inflammation), as the ensuing situation often cannot be alleviated with on-board treatment.

IV

Cardiopulmonary resuscitation on board

1 Cardiopulmonary resuscitation (CPR) on board commercial aircrafts

Sudden cardiac arrest has always a grim prognosis no matter where you are. Ultimately instant basic life support consisting of CPR (and defibrillation) is the only life saving measures – at least in some individuals. Thus, it is crucial to facilitate basic life support as early as possible wherever cardiac arrest occurs, even on board of commercial aircrafts.

All crews in commercial aviation are trained in basic life support and CPR. This includes the provision of oxygen as well as the application and use of fully automated defibrillators on board (AED). Even without professional medical support the necessary measures are initiated and carried out. Nevertheless, assistance of medical professionals is on board for all crews, especially in such a situation a great help.

Life-saving measurements will be provided until return of spontaneous circulation, death is declared or the passenger or patient, respectively, is handed over to ground ambulance providers.

During landing all passengers must be seated in upright position with belts securely fastened, thus CPR has to be interrupted. This is in the best interest of the safety of all passengers and crews on board. Only the captain may allow ongoing CPR, e.g. smooth landing maneuver anticipated.

2   Resuscitation procedures in general

Positioning of the patient

Neither aircraft seats nor the aisles provide enough space for initiation of CPR. Therefore the patient should be brought to a suitable location which can usually be found

- close to the galley with curtains facilitating at least some shelter or
- around the exit areas in wide body aircrafts.

Start CPR, get help and equipment

While initiating CPR

- call for assistance
- ask for medical equipment and AED
- notify cockpit crew

Usually one of the crew members coordinates the above mentioned aspects and keeps the cockpit crew informed to eventually reach out for a suitable diversion airport.

CPR – resuscitation procedures

Resuscitation is carried out following the ILCOR guidelines. Due to sufficient crew training the two person method is carried out and only interrupted to apply the AED or briefly during touchdown.

Automated external Defibrillator (AED)

The AED is utilized by flight attendants for resuscitation procedures following ILCOR and in Germany along the recommendations of the German Medical Association for early defibrillation by laypersons. The AED can only be discharged if the device recognizes ventricular fibrillation and recommends a shock. A shock discharge without this unambiguous recommendation by the AED, such as by a physician, is not possible.

Oxygen and drugs

Oxygen can be provided by a connector on the mask of the Ambu bag and can enrich ventilation with oxygen during resuscitation. The oxygen bottles on board provide a fix flow of 4 liters of oxygen per minute for 75 minutes (see Chapter I.4.3).

To enhance oxygen flow in spontaneous breathing patients the reservoir kit that comes with the Ambu bag in the Doctor's Kit can be utilized.

3 Resuscitation on board – Adults

CPR should always be applied following ILCOR guidelines as depicted on the following algorithm for Basic and Advanced Life Support (BLS or ALS). All crew members are trained at least once per year in the provision of BLS, including manoeuvres to place the patient in a suitable location on board of the aircraft. However, professional help from physicians, nurses or paramedics is highly appreciated.

Crew members, usually the purser, will also take care of structured communication with the cockpit. Recommendations from supporting physicians with regard to preferred diversion destinations or mandatory medical facilities on ground are always welcome, however, based on the crews' and all passengers safety the captain may not follow all advices.

Resuscitation with the AED – Basic life support by flight attendants

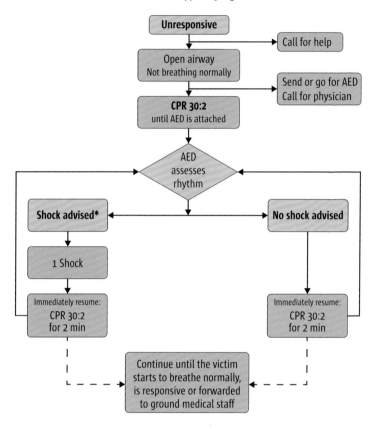

* Consider CPR 2 min before first shock (collapse > 4 min).
Compress chest at a rate of 100/min, change rescuers every 2 min, no check of pulse and breathing after shock.

Resuscitation with the AED – Advanced life support by physicians

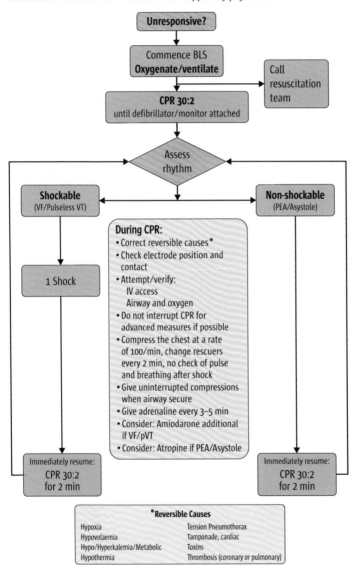

VF = Ventricular fibrillation; pVT = Pulseless ventricular tachycardia; PEA = Pulseless electrical activity

4 Resuscitation on board –
specific considerations for infants and children

In children and infants the cause of cardiac arrest is usually a disorder of respiratory function. In many cases simple basic maneuvers such as assisted breathing and/or ventilation with equipment, heart massage as well as supplemental oxygen may reestablish spontaneous circulatory function.

Resuscitation procedure is technically somewhat different in children and infants, please refer to the figures 33 to 36 and following algorithms.

For specific drug dosage in infants and children refer to table 10.

Although AED use is usually weigh restricted and not certified for human beings below 25 kg body weigh it can safely be applied in otherwise unsuccessful CPR.

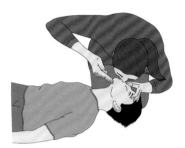

Fig. 33   Mouth-to-mouth ventilation on a child

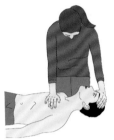

Fig. 34   Chest compressions with one hand on a child

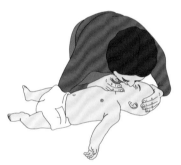

Fig. 35   Mouth-to-mouth ventilation on an infant

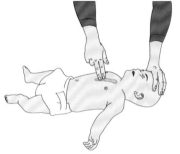

Fig. 36   Chest compressions on an infant

Tab. 10 Emergency dosage (IV) for children

	Dilution	Concentration	Dosage*	Infants	1 year old	6 years old	12 years old
Approx. weight				3 kg	10 kg	20 kg	40 kg
Adrenaline (1 mg/ml) **(diluted)**	1 Amp. + 9 ml NaCl 0.9%	0.01 mg/ml	0.01	0.3 ml	1.0 ml	2.0 ml	4.0 ml
Atropine (1 mg/ml)	n/a	1 mg/ml	0.01	0.06 ml	0.2 ml	0.4 ml	0.8 ml
Atropine (1 mg/ml) **(diluted)**	1 Amp. + 1 ml NaCl 0.9%	0.5 mg/ml	0.01	0.12 ml	0.44 ml	0.8 ml	1.6 ml
Amiodarone (150 mg/3 ml)	n/a	50 mg/ml	5	–	1 ml	2 ml	4 ml
Diazepam (10 mg/2 ml)	n/a	5 mg/ml	S: 0.07–0.15 C: 0.15–0.3	–	0.15–0.3 ml 0.3–0.6 ml	0.3–0.6 ml 0.6–1.2 ml	0.6–1.2 ml 1.2–2.4 ml
Midazolam (15 mg/3 ml)	n/a	5 mg/ml	S: 0.05 N: 0.15	–	0.1 ml 0.3 ml	0.2 ml 0.6 ml	0.4 ml 1.2 ml
Ketanest® S (50 mg/2 ml)	n/a	25 mg/ml	A: 0.125–0.25 N: 0.5–1.0	0.01–0.03 0.06–0.12	0.05–0.1 ml 0.2–0.4 ml	0.1–0.2 ml 0.4–0.8 ml	0.2–0.4 ml 0.8–1.6 ml

*in mg/kg body weight; S: sedation, C: anticonvulsant, N: narcotic, A: analgesic

Resuscitation with the AED (child) – Basic life support by flight attendants

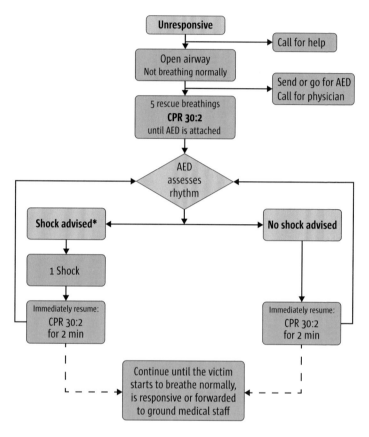

* Consider CPR 2 min before first shock (collapse > 4 min)

Resuscitation with the AED (Child) – Advanced life support by physicians

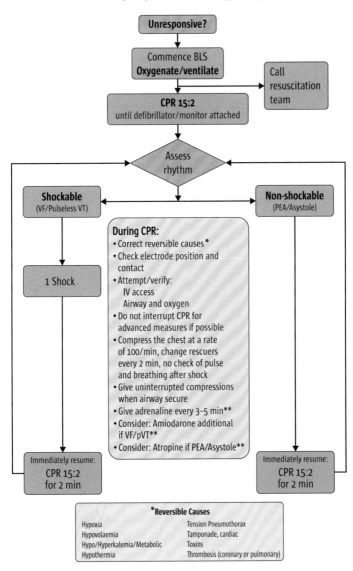

Unresponsive?

Commence BLS
Oxygenate/ventilate

Call
resuscitation
team

CPR 15:2
until defibrillator/monitor attached

Assess
rhythm

Shockable
(VF/Pulseless VT)

Non-shockable
(PEA/Asystole)

1 Shock

During CPR:
- Correct reversible causes *
- Check electrode position and
  contact
- Attempt/verify:
  IV access
  Airway and oxygen
- Do not interrupt CPR for
  advanced measures if possible
- Compress the chest at a rate
  of 100/min, change rescuers
  every 2 min, no check of pulse
  and breathing after shock
- Give uninterrupted compressions
  when airway secure
- Give adrenaline every 3–5 min**
- Consider: Amiodarone additional
  if VF/pVT**
- Consider: Atropine if PEA/Asystole**

Immediately resume:
CPR 15:2
for 2 min

Immediately resume:
CPR 15:2
for 2 min

*Reversible Causes	
Hypoxia	Tension Pneumothorax
Hypovolaemia	Tamponade, cardiac
Hypo/Hyperkalemia/Metabolic	Toxins
Hypothermia	Thrombosis (coronary or pulmonary)

** Dosage of medication due to weight;
VF = Ventricular fibrillation; pVT = Pulseless ventricular tachycardia; PEA = Pulseless electrical activity

V

Service/Appendix

1 Documentation of medical emergencies on board

There are emergency report forms in the Doctor's Kit and the First Aid Kit. The Emergency Report (see Fig. 37) facilitates and structures the documentation of an emergency event on board. All relevant data are requested in order to reconstruct the chronological process and the procedures undertaken. The report can be filled out by the assisting physician as well as employees and also serves to inform the ambulance personnel.

In the long run, the emergency reports help to improve the available medical equipment, when such determinations and measures are well documented.

Notfallprotokoll / Emergency Report

Medical Service

10 Flug-Nr. /Flight number:	14 Uhrzeit / Time (GMT):	16 Passagier / Passenger:	18 Geburtsdatum / Date of birth:	Passagier lehnt nach eingehender Aufklärung Behandlung ab. / Passenger refuses treatment after thorough advice.
11 Flug von / Flight from:	15 Name – PK Purser / Name – ID staff:	17 Heimatanschrift des Passagiers / Home address of the passenger:	19 Alter / Age:	
12 Flug nach / Flight to:			20 Geschlecht / Sex:	
			01 männlich / male	
			02 weiblich / female	
13 Datum / Date:				
	Unterschrift /Signature			Unterschrift / Signature of the passenger

Erstbefund / First Status

21 Ansprechbar / Conscious	01	Ja / Yes		02	Nein / No	
22 Puls / Pulse	01	Normal / Normal		02	Keinen / None	
	03	Schnell / Fast		04	Langsam / Slow	
23 Blutdruck / Blood Pressure	01	mmHg		02	Keinen / None	
24 Atmung / Breathing	01	Normal / Normal		02	Keine / None	
	03	Schnell / Fast		04	Schwer / Heavy	
25 Fieber / Fever	01	Ja / Yes		02	Nein / No	
26 Blass / Pale	01	Ja / Yes		02	Nein / No	
27 Kaltschweißig / Sweating	01	Ja / Yes		02	Nein / No	
28 Brustschmerz / Chest pain	01	Ja /Yes		02	Nein / No	
29 Kopfschmerz / Headache	01	Ja / Yes		02	Nein / No	
30 Verletzung / Injury	01	Ja / Yes		02	Nein / No	
31 Kopf / Head						
32 Arm / Arm						
33 Rumpf / Trunk						
34 Bein / Leg						
35 Vergiftung / Intoxication	01	Ja / Yes		02	Nein / No	
36 Alkohol / Alcohol						
37 Drogen / Drugs						
38 Sonstige / Other						

Behandlung / Treatment

39 Blutdruckmessung / Blood pressure check	
40 Sauerstoffgabe / Oxygen support	
41 Medizinische Untersuchung / Medical examination	
42 Venöser Zugang / Veinous access	
43 Medikation / Medication	
44 Atemwege frei / Airway restored	
45 Atemspende / Insufflation	
46 Intubation / Intubation	
47 Beatmung / Ventilation	
48 Reanimation / Resuscitation	
Erfolg / Success	
49 Wundversorgung / Wound care	
50 Verband / Bandage	
51 Schienung / Splint application	
52 AED-Benutzung / AED-Usage	
53 Defibrillation / Defibrillation	
Schockanzahl / Number of shocks:	
Erfolg / Success	
54 EKG-Monitoring / ECG-Monitoring	
55 SOS International Kontakt / SOS International Contact	
56 Telemedizin / Telemedicine Support	

Diagnose / Diagnosis

Herz-Kreislauf / Cardiovascular system		Atmung / Breathing		Ergebnis / Result	
57 Herz-Kreislauf / Cardiovascular system		62 Atmung / Breathing		67 Gesundheitszustand / Health condition	
01 Kreislaufkollaps / Circulatory collapse		01 Hyperventilation / Hyperventilation		01 Gebessert / Improved	
02 Brustschmerz / Chest pain		02 Asthmaanfall / Asthmatic attack		02 Unverändert / Unchanged	
03 Herzinfarkt / Myocardial infarction		03 Atemnot / Shortness of breath		03 Verschlechtert / Worsened	
04 Hochdruckkrise / Hypertensive crisis		04 Pneumonie / Pneumonia		04 Tot / Death	
58 Magen-Darm-Trakt / Gastrointestinal		05 Verschlucken-Bolus / Choking		68 Transport / Transportation	
01 Erbrechen / Vomiting		63 Stoffwechsel / Metabolism		01 Gehfähig / Able to walk	
02 Durchfall / Diarrhea		01 Unterzucker / Hypoglycemia		02 Rollstuhl / Wheelchair	
03 Kolik / Colic		02 Hyperglykämie / Hyperglycemia		03 Krankentrage / Stretcher	
Nieren / Kidney		03 Allergische Reaktion / Allergic reaction		69 Weiterbehandlung / Further treatment	
Gallenblase / Gallbladder		04 Alkoholmissbrauch / Alcohol abuse		01 Keine / None	
04 Akutes Abdomen / Acute abdomen		05 Vergiftung / Intoxication		02 Ambulant / Out-patient	
59 Schmerzen / Pain		64 Verletzungen / Injuries		03 Stationär / In-patient	
01 Kopfschmerz / Headache		01 Wunde / Wound		70 Flugverlauf / Flight progress	
02 Ohren / Ears		02 Blutung / Bleeding		01 Weiterflug / Continuation of flight	
03 Gelenke / Joints		03 Prellung / Contusion		02 Zwischenlandung / Diversion	
04 Sonstige / Other		04 Bruch / Fracture			
60 Nerven – Psyche / Neurologic – Psychiatric		05 Verbrühung / Scald			
01 Angststörung / Fear disorder		06 Verbrennung / Burn		Ziel / Destination:	
02 Unruhiger Passagier / Unruly Passenger		65 Gynäkologie / Gynecology			
03 Psychische Erkrankung / Mental illness		01 Geburt / Childbirth		71 Crew-Einsatzfähigkeit / Crew fit to fly	
04 Epileptischer Anfall / Seizures		02 Vaginalblutung / Vaginal bleeding		01 Ja / Yes	
05 Schlaganfall / Stroke		66 Sonstige Erkrankung / Other disease:		02 Nein / No	
61 Fieber – Infektion / Fever – Infection		01 Thrombose / Thrombosis			
		02 Lungenembolie / Lung embolism			

Bitte applizierte Medikation hier angeben / Please name the applied medication here:	Name des Arztes / Name of the doctor:
	Anschrift des Arztes / Address of the doctor:
Zusatzbemerkungen / Additional comments:	
	Unterschrift / Signature

Fig. 37 Emergency report form included in the First Aid Kit and Doctor's Kit

2 Doctor-On-Board programme

Physicians travelling on Lufthansa flights may be reluctant to volunteer during medical emergencies on board primarily because of insecurities regarding the conditions on board and because of legal aspects. In order to encourage them to assist during medical emergencies, Lufthansa German Airlines AG began a worldwide project in November 2006, called "Doctor On Board". All interested physicians have the option to register their medical specialty and thereby declare their willingness to assist in emergency situations. This registration is made online or by fax. The physician must provide a copy of the medical diploma and specialty certification. By assigning a code – there are six of them, for anaesthesiology, general medicine, internal medicine, gynaecology, neurology/psychiatry and one for miscellaneous specialties – the purser can then determine whether a physician is on board, where he or she is sitting and which field of specialization is represented. Obviously, there are no payments involved (see Chapter I.7), but rather a mileage certificate will be issued for each event, the amount of which is dependent on the circumstances. Upon registering, the physician receives a one-time certificate for 5,000 miles which is converted into a permanent card and is activated upon the first flight. For holders of Miles & More cards, the existing card is simply replaced by a new one with the corresponding code, and the initial 5,000 miles are put into the account after the first flight. This is in addition, of course, to the usual benefits of a Miles & More card.

With this card, a *network of interested physicians* is being built who are prepared to provide medical assistance for Lufthansa. Lufthansa will provide up-to-date information regarding procedures and equipment, and will attempt to increase the doctors' knowledge in this field with current training seminars.

The registration form is accessed through the *Lufthansa German Airlines AG* homepage http://www.lufthansa.com/us/en/Doctor-on-board. Registration details and contact information such as telephone and fax numbers are provided.

3 Lufthansa Medical Operation Center – worldwide unique

For those affected, any acute or chronic disease and physical or mental limitations may lead to restrictions of the so-called 'fitness to fly'. This can cause simple loss of comfort, affect one's health, or even jeopardize the safe operation of the flight for everyone involved. Often rather trivial issues such as dependency on chronic medication or insulin injections, restrictions with regard to sitting upright during taking off and landing, a cardiovascular or pulmonary risk assessment for the exposure to the cabin atmosphere (mild hypoxia), previous medical interventions or operations may sometimes require the assessment by an experienced flight surgeon.

An authoritative answer to all these questions is offered by the Medical Operation Center of Lufthansa (MOC), which – worldwide uniquely – is established into the medical service of Lufthansa and thereby serves as an interface on the one hand between medicine and flight operations, and on the other hand, between physicians or hospitals and passengers or patients.

The MOC advises and plans daily from 06:00 until 22:30 local time in Frankfurt/Germany air travel for acutely or chronically ill passengers, often on behalf of insurance or assistance companies as part of their repatriation procedure following illnesses or accidents aboard but also processes inquiries from hospitals, doctors or patients themselves. All MOC staff are trained medical specialists with diverse medical backgrounds (e.g. as a nurse, paramedic, elder care, medical practitioner, midwife) and have an additional training in the field of aviation industries (travel professionals, ticket agents, care service, cabin crew, flight manager), so that the medical challenge can be included into the regulatory and logistical processes of flight operations. Thus, the MOC serves as an interface for both, the medical as well as the logistical aspects of planning and implementation of patient repatriation.

Various medical and organizational support options are available for scheduled air services based on the needs and/or indication of the customers or patients, such as supplemental oxygen (Wenoll system), extra leg space/room for leg elevation, lying transportation on a stretcher (always supported technically by a nurse, paramedic or doctor). This may also involve – again, a MOC uniqueness, but limited here to long-haul fleets only – intensive care transport which means utilizing the Patient Transport Compartment (PTC).

Regardless of the medical or organizational challenges, a safe flight and a correspondingly safe and comfortable patient transport is in most cases feasible. In case of doubt or complex medical problems, a doctor-to-doctor conversation is possible at any time.

The Medical Operation Center can be contacted at +49 69 696 55077 or medicaloperation@dlh.de, daily from 06:00 until 22:30 local time in Frankfurt/Germany.

4 Recommended literature

Blettner M, Zeeb H, Langner I, Hammer G: Epidemiologische Studie beim fliegenden Personal der Deutschen Lufthansa und der LTU. Dt. Ärzteblatt 99: 51–52, A-3462 / B-2918 / C-2718, Köln 2002

Cocks R, Liew M: Commercial aviation in-flight emergencies and the physician. Emerg Med Australas 2007; 19(1): 1–8

Curdt-Christiansen C, Draeger J, Kriebel J (Hrsg.): Principles and Practice Of Aviation Medicine. World Scientific, Singapore, 2009

Davis JR, Johnson R, Stepanek J, Fogarty JA (Hrsg.): Fundamentals of Aerospace Medicine. 4. Auflage, Lippincott Williams & Wilkins, Philadelphia, 2008

Dietel M, Suttorp N, Zeitz M (2012) Harrisons Innere Medizin. 18. Auflage, ABW Wissenschaftsverlag, Berlin, 2012

Draeger J, Kriebel J (Hrsg.): Praktische Flugmedizin. Ecomed Verlagsgesellschaft, Landsberg/Lech, 2002

Egerth M, Pump S, Graf J: Aviation and high-altitude medicine for anaesthetists – Part 4: Human Performance Limitations and Crew Resource Management. Anasthesiol Intensivmed Notfallmed Schmerzther 2013; 48: 424–428

Graf J, Stüben U, Pump S: Aviation and high-altitude medicine for anaesthetists - Part 3: Emergencies on board commercial aircrafts. Anasthesiol Intensivmed Notfallmed Schmerzther 2013; 48: 224–229

Graf J, Seiler O, Pump S, Günther M, Albrecht R: Aviation and high-altitude medicine for anaesthetists – Part 2: Long-haul intensive care transports. Anasthesiol Intensivmed Notfallmed Schmerzther 2013; 48: 76–82

Graf J, Stüben U, Pump S: In-flight medical emergencies. Dtsch Arztebl Int 2012; 109: 591–602

Graf J, Stüben U: Notfall an Bord von Flugzeugen – was steht zur Verfügung, was kann ich tun, was darf ich tun? Kardiologie up2date 2012; 8: 114–123

von Hintzenstern U (Hrsg.): Notarzt-Leitfaden. 6. Auflage, Urban & Fischer, München, 2010

Houston S, Graf J, Sharkey J: Commercial air travel after intraocular gas injection. Aviat Space Environ Med 2012 Aug;83(8): 809–10

Hung KKC, Chan EYY, Cocks RA, Ong RM, Rainer TH, Graham CA: Predictors of flight diversions and death for in-flight medical emergencies in commercial aviation. Arch Intern Med 2010; 170: 1401–1402

Kretschmer H, Kusch G, Scherbaum H: Reisemedizin. 2. Auflage, Urban & Fischer, München, 2005

Küpper T, Rieke B, Muth C-M (Hrsg.): Moderne Reisemedizin, Gentner Verlag, Stuttgart, 2013

Müller S: Memorix Notfallmedizin. 9. Auflage, Thieme Verlag, Stuttgart, 2011

Muhm JM, Rock PB, McMullin DL, Jones SP, Lu IL, Eilers KD, Space DR, McMullen A: Effect of aircraft-cabin altitude on passenger discomfort. N Engl J Med. 2007; 357(1):18–27

Nicolai T: Pädiatrische Notfall- und Intensivmedizin. 4. Auflage, Springer Verlag, Berlin, Heidelberg, 2011

Nolan JP, Soar J, Cariou A, Cronberg T, Moulaert VR, Deakin CD, Bottiger BW, Friberg H, Sunde K, Sandroni C: European Resuscitation Council and European Society of Intensive Care Medicine Guidelines for Post-resuscitation Care 2015: Section 5 of the European Resuscitation Council Guidelines for Resuscitation 2015. Resuscitation 2015. Oct. 15 Vol. 95. 202-22. URL: http://www.resuscitationjournal.com/article/S0300-9572%2815%2900330-5/fulltext (abgerufen am 25.01.16)

Pump S, Stüben U, Graf J: Aviation and high-altitude medicine for anaesthetists – Part 1: Physical basics and pathophysiology. Anasthesiol Intensivmed Notfallmed Schmerzther 2012;47(11–12): 682–7

Rainford DJ, David P. Gradwell DP (Hrsg.): Ernsting's Aviation and Space Medicine. 5th ed. CRC Press, Boca Raton, FL [u.a.], 2014

Scholz J, Sefrin P, Böttinger B (et al., Hrsg.): Notfallmedizin. 3. Auflage, Thieme Verlag, Stuttgart, 2012

Sefrin P, Schua R: HEXAL Notfall Manual. 7. Auflage, Urban & Fischer, München, 2012

Shrikrishna D, Coker RK: Air Travel Working Party of the British Thoracic Society Standards of Care Committee Managing passengers with stable respiratory disease planning air travel: British Thoracic Society recommendations. Thorax 2011; 66(9): 831–833

Silverman D, Gendreau M: Medical issues associated with commercial flights. Lancet 2009; 373(9680): 2067–2077

Smith D, Toff, W, Joy M: Fitness to fly for passengers with cardiovascular disease. Heart 2010; 96 Suppl 2: ii1–16

Tonks A: Cabin fever. BMJ 2008; 336(7644): 584–586

Watson HG, Baglin TP: Guidelines on travel-related venous thrombosis. Br J Haematol 2011; 152(1):31–34

Weber R, Kühnel T, Graf J, Hosemann W. Aerosinusitis. Teil 1: Grundlagen, Pathophysiologie und Prophylaxe. HNO 2014; 62 (1): 57–64

Weber R, Kühnel T, Graf J, Hosemann W. Aerosinusitis. Teil 2: Diagnostik, Therapie und Wiederaufnahme der Flugtätigkeit. HNO 2014; 62 (2): 297–306

Index

Emergency index

Index